"Americans urgently need to know more about every aspect of the destruction wrought by illicit drugs.

"*Addicted* offers sorely needed information from the front lines, [shedding] light on adolescents as addicts.

"In their own words, 10 youngsters describe how they spun out of control, starting with early experimentation with alcohol and marijuana (most were younger than 13 when they began), to a point where, in the words of one youth, they 'just couldn't relate to anything except drugs.'

"Their backgrounds include both strict and permissive families. One is struck by how often these youngsters talk of divorce and physical abuse, of foster care and adoption, of shyness and a sense of not fitting in, and of the enormous pleasure they experienced from their first tastes of alcohol and drugs.

"The inside look we are offered is illuminating and gripping. Joel Engel's interviews contribute to our understanding of drug using."

— *The New York Times*

# ADDICTED

## In Their Own Words: Kids Talking about Drugs as told to Joel Engel

**Foreword by Michael L. Peck, Ph.D.**

TOR®

A TOM DOHERTY ASSOCIATES BOOK
NEW YORK

ADDICTED
IN THEIR OWN WORDS: KIDS TALKING ABOUT DRUGS



A Tor Book
Published by Tom Doherty Associates, Inc.
49 West 24th Street
New York, N.Y. 10010

Cover design by Joe Curcio

ISBN: 0-812-59446-7

First edition: August 1989
First mass market printing: May 1990

Printed in the United States of America

0 9 8 7 6 5 4 3 2 1

Thanks to Susan Finch at the Clare Foundation in Santa Monica, California, and Angela Wosyk at I-ADARP, Inc., in Van Nuys, California, for their guidance and assistance. And special thanks to all the kids.

# ADDICTED

# Foreword

The year 1988 marks the twenty-fifth year, a quarter of a century, since the drug-abuse plague was unleashed upon the United States. It was in 1963 that from the hallowed halls of Harvard came the pronouncements by Professors Leary and Alpert that LSD was a wonder drug. It was seen in those days of the early sixties, particularly by college students, as a potential cure for alcoholism and mental illness, a mind-expanding, benign substance that would create peace and harmony in the world, reduce violence, and enhance one's creative powers. This is a far cry, we can see, from the world revealed by the stories in this book. The despair, the desperation, the pain—all the suffering and hopelessness that accompany drug and alcohol use—were not foretold by the early "prophets of acid."

As the sixties progressed, we saw LSD, marijuana, cocaine, amphetamines, barbiturates, and, of course, the ever-present alcohol used in a wide variety of settings, particularly on college campuses and in college-oriented communities. Toward the end of the sixties, we witnessed the influx of many of these drugs into high school communities, and by the early seventies, we had seen outbreaks and epidemics of hard drugs, such as heroin, in middle-class suburban communities. The plague continued throughout the seventies—a plague in a sense every bit as virulent, deadly, tragic as the bubonic plague of the Middle Ages, and one which was probably responsible for more deaths. Drug use and alcohol abuse were widespread in high schools by the middle seventies and in junior high schools by the late seventies. Early in the next decade, it was not uncommon to hear about children age ten or eleven using marijuana, drinking heavily, and even moving on to cocaine. Children whose bodies and minds had not even moved into puberty were already poisoning their bodies. Then, in about the middle eighties, we began to see some breathing room. We began to see some hope in the battle against the great drug plague. Alcohol was still in use by a large portion of the teenage population. Cocaine was being used more frequently than ever before, although still in the two-to-four-percent range by teenagers. But marijuana use was down. Use of other dangerous drugs such as speed, downers, and PCP, was down, even though the use of LSD and mushrooms had made a comeback in the eighties. There was a general trend away from drug use and abuse and a strong anti-drug movement among teenagers: to say No to drugs, to recover from drugs, and to fight the plague.

My own interest in alcohol and drug use, particularly among teenagers, dates back to the sixties, when I began my research and clinical work in teen suicide. Having continued that work for the last twenty years, I have seen teen suicide slowly increase to the present-day "epidemic" proportions in correlation with the rise of alcohol and drug use in teenagers, particularly as younger and younger teens became enamored of and then addicted to alcohol and drugs. Today most research suggests that about half of all teens who commit suicide, and approximately that many of those who attempt suicide, are chemically dependent. We're not talking about people who have a sip of beer on Saturday night or take a hit on a joint once a month. We're talking about people who are heavily involved in alcohol and drugs, much like the people who tell their stories in this book. As you read these stories, you'll see for yourself how frequently the word "suicide" comes up in many different contexts and from many different youngsters who might otherwise have never dreamed the word.

Another horrible and even more frequent cause of death among teenagers is traffic accidents. The carnage on our highways has been horrendous, and close to fifty percent of those teens who have lost their lives have been identified as driving under the influence or as being killed by someone driving under the influence. But the number of those teens who are not clearly identified as drunk, but who were driving and dying on LSD, cocaine, marijuana, or a variety of other mind-altering substances, is unknown. The provisions for testing for this vary from state to state and from jurisdiction to jurisdiction. The numbers may well be beyond fifty percent. We can fairly accurately foretell that about 2500 of the teenagers who die of suicide each year have been under the influence of alcohol or drugs. Many times that number die on the highways under the influence of alcohol or drugs. But there is yet another unmentioned source of death, destruction, and misery, and that is homicide. Another two or three thousand young people are murdered each year, and often alcohol or drugs are involved.

So far, we have been talking about thousands of young people dying each year as a result of accidents, suicide, and homicide where alcohol and drugs have been a major contributing factor. But we haven't begun to touch the survivors, the burnouts, the emotional basket cases, the ruined lives, the pain, the carnage, the destruction of families and friends. This book is as good as or better than any other at telling those stories. Here you'll find the stories of some innocent teens, boys and girls next door, who rapidly moved down the path of destruction, who wasted and trashed much of their lives, who wound up on the edge of suicide. You'll see some teens who have a long history of alcohol or drug abuse in their family. In these cases the family alcoholism or drug use, past or present, played a major role in pointing the young people toward the path of self-destruction. You'll see the twisted, tortured, distorted perceptions, the damaged judgments, the apathy, and most of all the wasted lives over and over again as you read each story. You'll be struck by the waste, the horrible waste, of each precious life. Even those teens who don't attempt suicide, who don't die, have in common that same depressing apathy, and make the same depressing statement: "I really didn't care if I lived or died."

Sometimes these stories become difficult to read. Sometimes you'll feel as though "I just don't want to read about that much pain." Yet there's a fascination, a feeling of being drawn to the next paragraph and the next page, a feeling of anticipation, of hoping that the person telling the story has recovered, put it behind him or her, survived. And as you read each story and experience each struggle for survival, the sad thought will recur: "So many of these children don't survive. What can we do about that?"

I think this book is a contribution to that cause. If enough of us read about, feel, and understand the pain, the struggle, and the tragic waste of these children, maybe we'll all do just a little bit more.

Michael L. Peck, Ph.D.
Director, Suicide Prevention Center
Los Angeles, California
October 1987

# Introduction

"War Stories" is the term that young people sometimes use to describe their experiences with drugs. Like old soldiers, the kids sit and swap tales. Unlike the soldiers, they do so without bragging; while the drugs have certainly taken a toll on their bodies, the wounds are mostly psychic, and "topping" someone means detailing more degradation and despair.

The accounts included here are all true. Except for deleting many of the "you knows" and "likes" which punctuate kids' speech and organizing what were often jumbled, incomplete, and/or confusing thoughts into a coherent narrative, the stories are presented exactly as the kids told them—in their own words.

I met these kids, ages fifteen to twenty-one, through rehabilitation agencies all over southern California. I explained to the directors and counselors what I was looking for: kids willing to share their experiences in a forthright and honest manner. Originally I had intended to tell the stories of kids who were still using, but I quickly learned that they were either unwilling or unable to tell the truth, and that only kids who had admitted their addictions and sought help would speak truthfully.

The interviews, which took place between August of 1986 and April of 1987, were conducted at the various rehab houses, in small, depressing rooms that smelled permanently of stale tobacco smoke and echoed with the sounds of the traffic on adjacent streets and alleys. The kids and I sat opposite each other on frayed upholstery that someone had probably donated after a lifetime of use, or on aluminum and plastic chairs bought with limited funds.

In all, ten stories were selected for this collection. Though a number of other kids were interviewed, their narrations were hopelessly convoluted. In every case, I omitted any geographical references. These kids come from every area of the country. They represent all economic, racial, and religious backgrounds and have in common only that they went through rehab in southern California. All of them were trying desperately to anesthetize themselves against pain, both real and imagined.

When I undertook this assignment, I believed that I would be able to discern some reason which might explain why one person can merely experiment with drugs, while another becomes addicted; moreover, I wanted to know what factors drive kids to use drugs in the first place. While there were some recurring themes—peer pressure, divorce, shyness, isolation, parental abuse—these commonalities seemed bound by the thinnest of threads, and it would reduce each individual's experience to a cliché to pretend that any of these circumstances, by itself or in tandem, was responsible. In the end, tidy answers and explanations lead only to more questions.

Listening to the kids tell their stories, I often became speechless. I kept thinking of myself at their age—how different my life was and how much older, in some ways, they seemed. Drug addiction is a horror I had been exposed to before, but never in such young people. Somehow, the destruction that drugs and alcohol inflict seems so much more appalling in those who have their whole lives ahead of them.

No matter how gruesome the details, the kids always spoke candidly—not as a catharsis, but as a gentle warning. Although they are reluctant to proselytize, believing that everyone must make his or her own decisions about whether to use, they are glad to share the truths that they discovered, through experience, about drugs and drug addiction.

Ultimately, these are stories of hope and joy. After years of self-hatred, these kids have come to like themselves;

they are sober (in every case but two they have remained clean since the interviews; the fact that two could not maintain sobriety does not debunk their stories, but emphasizes how difficult addiction is to break) and they are alive. And at least for now, that's good enough.

Joel Engel
Topanga, California
May 1987

# ALLEN

**"Once it happens and it's got you in its motherfuckin' grip, there ain't nothing you can do, 'cause then it's all about ball and chain."**

My parents are the kind of people that can make a gallon of wine last a year long. Not me. When I was nine or ten, even, I was tryin' to cop a buzz. At family parties I'd go around and finish off people's drinks and stuff like that. They'd give me a tiny glass of wine, and I thought it looked real adult, real mature, to be able to drink with everyone. And I always wanted more and more and more, and I never seemed to get enough. Right from day one. I remember one of my first drinking experiences was in sixth grade with this guy named Cory. He had decided to spend the night at my house. I was a real crazy little sixth grader, and I remember I ended up goin' downstairs to get into my mom's liquor cabinet when they were sleeping. And I remember finishing off this bottle of Cutty Sark, and Cory downed a little too much and threw up all over the place. That experience still kind of stands out in my mind because I, you know, I began to enjoy it. That was, like, the first time actually sneaking a drink.

Allen, twenty when he was interviewed for this book, comes from an upper-middle-class family. When he received straight A's through the sixth grade, his parents had no reason to assume he would turn out any differently from his older sisters, both of whom became respected professionals married to other respected professionals.

My parents are extremely conservative. They'd, you know, told me about certain kids in the neighborhood who I, quote-unquote, shouldn't hang around with, and being myself real rowdy and real rambunctious, I said, "Hmm, well let's see what they want me to stay away from." So I met this guy, Chris, and he ended up introducing me to pot. I remember I smoked pot for the first time and I walked in the house, and this was after a huge fight with my parents, and I was all stoned, and I just felt great. I don't think I necessarily went out to get high just because I had a fight with my parents that time, but it seemed, you know, like a good time to do it; I went out basically for curiosity: Just what is it, why does everybody do this, and why does everybody say stay away from it?

I don't come from a, quote-unquote, broken home or anything like that. My parents were completely normal. Yeah, real normal. I sometimes got along with them, but it was like, basically, they always tried to have control over me, and make me the way they wanted me to be. And just the way I am, I rebelled from day one. I'm not saying that I wouldn't have tried pot anyway, because I would have. I would have found out about it and used it whether they tried to keep me away from it or not. After I started partying all the time, my grades just went straight downhill, and my parents couldn't figure out why. They didn't have a clue.

When his grades slipped, Allen was enrolled in a private school for academically gifted children who fail to live up to their potentials. He did well for a short time there, away from his old friends, but when the old pattern began to emerge, sometime around the seventh grade, he was placed in what his parents thought was a much stricter boarding school in another state.

That school was my first introduction to people who had been partying a long time and people who'd been through the jail systems, etcetera, and so on. I don't know, for some reason that really attracted me—the people that were the diehards, so to speak. The people who were crazy, you know, who just absolutely had a real nutty aspect on things, real crazy, who were fightin' all the time, and partying down all the time, who just basically just didn't give a fuck. For some reason, that just hit home with me. I guess it's just my nature. To say the least, I ended up learning a lot from these people, like as far as street ways and listening to things, and about fighting and the whole bit. I started, you know, to shape my life around everything, around all that stuff, and then I stayed there about six months, and then I went to a school over in . . . [an adjacent state].

That was really great. The school was absolutely out of control. My first day there I remember partying. It was like I never had too much time to experiment with drugs 'cause I never knew anybody who had any, but once I got into that school, it was like all these drugs became completely available to me. I started hangin' around with a partying crowd, and I knew the talk and I knew the walk. I was just turning thirteen. There was one kind of pill that I took when I was there that they were afraid I was gonna overdose on. Approximately six people had taken this Saudi Arabian drug called Artaine—it's over-the-counter there. It was, to say the least, a real hard hallucinogenic. It was like a hallucinogenic and a painkiller together in a pill form. And I remember eatin' about four of these things and just seein' all kinds of absolutely bizarre shit on these drugs. The people that'd taken it before I had taken it were seeing, like, killer rats and stuff like that, and we had just gotten back from Christmas vacation, and they were already packed up and ready to go on Christmas vacation—they were so mixed up.

By this time the adults there were checkin' everybody's eyes in the whole camp to see who else was on it. And they came into my room around twelve at night on the day I took it for the first and only time. The way I got it was, I had explained to this guy who was selling it that I had a backache and needed something for the pain. I said, "Fuck, I wouldn't mind takin' a few of these Artaine, you know, they look pretty stoney." So he gave me a handful—I don't remember how many. I took the whole handful and popped 'em in my mouth and swallowed 'em just like that with a glass of water, and you know, and it seemed fine to me, and hours later, things started happenin' real radically—seein' all kinds of stuff, boy. Then I passed out. They woke me up to check my eyes. Somebody could say a sentence to me and I couldn't repeat the first word of it unless I'd hear it about ten or eleven times. And after, after that period of time I'd—a lot of people told me I'd really screwed myself up. I remember my memory was horrible for about the next six months. I was real slow in speaking. I only took it that once.

That experience was my first big step up from pot. That was, like, moving my way up the scale. Next thing after that was black beauties—you know, speed. I'd started taking those every once in a while. A girl who was there used to get 'em every once in a while. Her friends used to send 'em to her in stuffed animals. I used to every once in a while buzz up and down the school. That was pretty wild. I didn't sleep hardly at all. My appetite at that time was gone. I started to become real skinny.

At fourteen, Allen was brought back to live at home with his parents, who soon saw that he was beyond their control. They decided that he needed discipline and told him they planned to send him to another boarding school.

I told 'em flat out, they could go and rot somewhere 'cause I wasn't gonna go back to school and was nobody gonna force me. And so I started comin' in drunk. I'd finally discovered Quaaludes at this time. Quaaludes and vodka. I thought it was an absolutely bitchin' combination. I mean, I'm tellin' you, I used to, you know—I remember riding home on a few different occasions, running into mailboxes and parked cars on my bicycle and just gigglin' my ass off, and it was, you know, it was kind of real sad 'cause I remember just comin' in and barely bein' able to make it up the stairs to finally hit my bed and knock right out.

My parents knew I was out of control, and there was nothin' they could do. Absolutely nothing. To say the least, at that time they didn't have much training on alcoholism or anything else, so they ended up finally—I just woke up one morning and I remember sittin' in bed and four big guys come walkin' in my room. They said, "Hello, we're from . . . [a reformatory in a Western state] and you're coming with us." And I said, "Fuck that. You guys ain't takin' me nowhere." And I took a swing and hit one guy in the mouth, you know, and he kinda lurched back, and the next thing I know they'd flipped me over and had me handcuffed, and I took a bite out of this guy's leg. They had me kickin' and screamin', goin' out, you know, and I remember being shoved in my mother's car next to this one guy with no neck, who later on turned out to be my therapist. I used to call him "No Neck" because his shoulders were so high up it almost looked like he had no neck.

My mom came over to the window of the car and said, "I'm sorry it had to be this way," and this, that, and the other. And at that point, when that started to happen, such a hate inside myself began to burn for her, for my dad, it was incredible. Just, "I'm gonna kill 'em when I get out, I'm gonna kill 'em!" And she came over to the window and said she was sorry, and I said, "Bitch, when I get out you'll get yours," and I spit in her face, you know, and she just went sobbing off in tears, just totally losing it.

They threw me on an airplane and I was taken in handcuffs to this school, where they shaved my head and dressed me in pink fluorescent pajamas and gave me a minimum of 200 hours to stand and stare at a white brick wall. You got two hours off for every one hour you stood looking at this wall. If you didn't stare at the wall there was always the thing called the "pee room," where they'd toss you in a little cubicle about seven feet high, about five feet long, and about four feet wide, with this steel door, and they wouldn't let you out to go to the bathroom. That's why they called it the "pee room." They'd toss you in there and let you think about it for a while. You'd stay in there depending on when your attitude got better. Until you were willin' to do what they told you to do. Several hours, several days, you know, they'd feed you and the whole bit, but it wasn't too pleasant.

My attitude always remained real good when I was at this place. I wasn't defiant. When I got there I just said, "Well, I'll do what they ask me to do." I was scared, you know, I was tryin' to figure out what was goin' on. You know, I'm in these pink fluorescent pajamas starin' at this goddamn white brick wall, with no hair, goin', "What the fuck?" I don't think I deserved what was being done to me. I don't think anybody deserves that. I don't think I'd waste that kind of shit on my worst enemy. I spent two years there with their, quote-unquote, rehabilitative therapy. It was a total-lockdown kind of place. Just like prison. Only in prison you can get drugs. Since I was off the drugs, I excelled in academics like crazy. I was gettin' straight A's. I took all the classes and passed every class with flying colors. The classwork was pretty easy, and after a while I began to know everyone there, and pretty soon, towards the end of my stay, I didn't have to go to class and I learned how to clean the pool. And all I did there, you know, was just work out and spar with some buddies of mine. We'd raise hell every once in a while, you know, and end up on incident report and have to stand so many hours in front of the wall. But nothing too bad.

I remember when I finally came to the day, you know, when I could leave. I couldn't believe I was goin'. It'd been two years. It was an all-boys school, so I hadn't seen a girl in two years. I had just turned about sixteen. I was so infuriated that I'd spent two years there. Yeah. I'd engraved that in my soul. There was nothing but the entire payback on my mind for the whole two years—to get back at my parents. I figured I'd just spent two years of my life because of you assholes, now I'm gonna do something to you!

They treated me real different when I got back. It was like, "Oh, we haven't seen you in two years and this that and the other, it's nice you're well now," and treatin' me like a sicko and the whole bit, and I just disrespected them from day one. You know, right from the minute I got off the airplane I said, the first thing, "I need a fuckin' dollar and a quarter for a pack of cigarettes," and they couldn't believe it. I'd gotten out there, doing so well and everything, they were shocked.

Allen attended a public high school near his parents' home. He no longer had any friends in the area and made new ones slowly. In time, though, he got acquainted with "a partying crowd." His unwavering motivation remained getting even with his parents.

I met some, quote-unquote, longhairs and the burners and everything else. Stoners, just burnout people. You know, those people were smokin' a lot of dope and doin' acid and shit like that. And I started to, at that point in time, quote-unquote, pay my parents back. I knew the things to say and do that would hurt them. We were startin' to get in fights again, and they all, you know, they couldn't figure out what was goin' on.

I'd finally gotten a new pot connection. I was drinking a little, you know, here and there, not too much. And finally I decided, well, you know, what'll be a good initial payback, and by this time I'd started to meet enough people to where I had a good set of, you know, friends. Now, a lot of these people were heroin junkies, people who were shootin' dope, rowdies. Some of the older people weren't in high school but friends of the people I went to high school with. And at this point in time I ended up rippin' off my parents blind. I went in and stole a bunch of my dad's expensive stuff, like a big old coin collection worth thousands and thousands of dollars. I hocked it off for a few hundred bucks. You know, I didn't really care how much I got just as long as I got back at them. Everything I did, basically, was to get back at them. Yeah. Everything. I stole just basically about everything: silverware, mink coats, checks, credit cards, the whole run-through. At that point in time it wasn't really to get money for dope. But later on, about four months down the road after getting out, I'd finally started hanging around people who were doin' a lot of coke, and I ended up with a lot of money one day from hockin' off a bunch of these coins. I got my first coke, and I rapid-fired right through that. You know, just went right through it like it wasn't even there. I fuckin' enjoyed it so much, you know, went out and got more and more. And after that I was no longer stealing from my parents to get back—it was all about supporting my habit.

My parents knew what I was doing, but I guess they figured that the reformatory thing obviously wasn't gonna do anything for me after two years of being out there, and obviously nothing else was gonna change once they put me back out there. I guess they didn't know what to do. Other than call the police, which is what they did later.

I went from snorting coke to basing to shooting coke within probably about a period of two weeks. And at that point, I finally came across heroin, which is, you know—it goes along with coke, hand in hand. It's a short step, especially if you're shootin' coke. And I discovered when you mix the two together, boy, you get one hell of a feeling.

Finally my parents called up the police and I was arrested. They told them that I'd been stealing from them and using drugs, and I was busted for grand larceny. I woke up, once again, to two cops, who handcuffed me, took me down, fingerprinted me, photographed me, and sent me off to juvenile hall, which, to say the least, I kind of liked. It didn't really bother me, you know. It was real easy in there. If somebody gave me a hard time I could just stand up and hit him in the mouth, you know—somebody's givin you a bad time, just book him, yeah. I'd spent a lot of time learning how to fight. That was something that really appealed to me, to be able to get out my aggression on someone's face. And so anyway, I ended up goin' over to this place, some kind of drug-dependency center. I stayed in there for about two weeks and basically told them what they could do with their program and their style of living. I told them to fuck off and I split. I just walked right out. Ran out the front door. I was still sixteen at the time.

Allen's parents, in a desperate panic, knowing that he cared little or nothing about himself and others, went through legal channels to have him committed to a mental institution—where it turned out to be easy to score drugs. After six months, the time to which he was sentenced by the courts, he was back out on the streets.

This time, it was, you know, it was all about that first fix. I figured, I got this comin! You know, and I got back out and started up again, only this time I'd met a guy, Phil, who right now is over in Folsom State Prison doin' a little time. But anyway, what happened was he taught me the great art of robbing houses. And after that, me and him became, you know, team one, 'cause I basically had a good knowledge. I'd done a lot of reading and knew a lot of things about drugs, like the PDR [Physician's Desk Reference] and different drug books and different kinds of drugs and different tests to tell what's what and what's in what. Basically I'd learned about every drug in detail: how to test it, you know, what's good, what isn't. I always had an available connection. So it was like I started robbin' these houses and we would hit . . . [two well-to-do areas about thirty miles apart]. I mean, just ransacking all these wealthy houses. We were making two thousand dollars a day. We'd rent out a hotel room and buy a bunch of cocaine and some heroin and end up shootin' up all night.

There was a lot of people that we used to know to sell the stolen stuff to. There was one guy in the Mafia that we used to know that—he used to, shall we say, give us addresses of people who owed him. He used to give us addresses and we used to casually go out and hit up these houses, and he'd say, "Well, I want this, this, and this, and you can keep this and this." That went on for a while. You just kept goin' and, you know, things just slowly but surely started to pick up. I started shootin' more and more and more heroin all the time—I was a full-blown junkie by now. I was living at home, or in a hotel room, stealing all this merchandise to support my habit from houses all over, with some crazy-ass dude following me. This detective, a cop, had found out about me. He'd found out about me 'cause, you know, from the first time I ripped off a house, somebody had dropped a name, and it just happened to have been mine. So this cop had been trailin' me a long time, and me and Phil, to say the least, were doing quite well. Because we would leave no footprints, no fingerprints, it would always look like the entrance was done with a passkey. One of our, quote-unquote, burglar trademarks was to go in there and, if you felt hungry, make yourself some lunch, and if the person had any dope, shoot all their dope in their kitchen and leave the works there and just split.

I did a lot of reading in a lot of different libraries, and talked with a lot of people in the, quote-unquote, field of professional robbery. And I learned how to rewire a lot of alarms; how to get through a lot of systems in a lot of different ways, you know, and there were different techniques of, like, clipping three wires and, like, clipping the ground wire and connecting all three of them together. The alarm would go off for a second, but when you connected all the wires back together it would seem like somebody went in the house, the alarm went off, and they'd turned off the alarm, which would mean they were the owner. So nothing would happen.

I had done armed robberies, but I was never caught. I didn't like the feeling I got from the whole ordeal. To say the least, I kinda was shittin' bricks half the time; it wasn't real fun. You know, if somebody came home, I always had two exits. I always knew two ways to get the fuck out of that house, so I was not caught. If somebody, I think, if somebody would've caught me I would've probably beaten 'em down or shot 'em. You know, 'cause I knew what to do, I knew how to handle myself. I usually carried a gun. If it came down to my life or theirs, I wasn't gonna die. I don't think I really cared about whether I lived or died, you know, I just cared about scoring and hittin' up. That was my whole life. I really didn't, you know, to say the least, I didn't care too much about myself. I didn't. I didn't give a flying fuck. I was livin' in my parents' house, and we never even talked to each other. Sometimes my mom or dad would walk in my room when I was fixin' up, and they'd see the needle hangin' out my arm, and they'd just turn around and walk back out.

Usually I'd stay way the fuck away from my own neighborhood. I wouldn't rob houses in my neighborhood 'cause it's bad news. But finally I figured, well, my neighborhood's extremely rich, and I know all the places that have all the dough and the safes and everything else. Easy to pick money. So I went on a fuckin' big old spree up there, huge spree. Yeah. Neighbors just went wild, 'cause they couldn't figure out what was going on. Ten, eleven, fifteen houses were getting robbed a day. And nobody, nobody could figure out what was happenin'.

I'd go door to door and I'd get to the end of the block and I'd carry a pad with me and I'd ring doorbells. You know, "Hello, is such and such home? Oh, they don't live at this address? Damn I'm sorry." And this guy'd point this place out. "The address is right here." And I mean, if nobody was home, I'd write down the address. By the time I got to the end of the block I'd have five addresses written down and I'd just go back and clean out the places, you know, end up carrying all this stuff to the end of the street. And usually in the last house I'd make a phone call to a friend and have him just drop by the corner and pick me up with all the shit. Sometimes there was so much stuff I couldn't carry all of it. Usually I had to ditch half or three-quarters of it because it was so heavy. You know, I'd end up with so much silverware, after a while, it gets a little heavy, and especially when you got these twenty-four-place-setting silver sets worth thousands and thousands of dollars. I'm doin' this, basically, you know, for my habit, and the thrill and the adventure, I think, were kind of in there. I don't think I was tryin' to get back at my parents anymore, though. Mostly it was my habit. I was usually doin' about four, five bags of heroin a day and all the cocaine I could buy.

Still not eighteen, Allen continued to rob houses to support his habit, even after his first partner and then a second one were busted and sent to prison.

Seein' those guys get nailed should've told me something, but being the kind of person I was, I didn't listen, even to myself. So I just started working with this other partner, this guy I'd known for a long time who would tell me he was, you know, robbin' houses for a long time—a, quote-unquote, pro. So I remember I robbed one house with this guy and we got chased down the street by the owners, and I knew this guy's obviously a fool. I said, "Uh-uh, I shouldn't be workin' with this guy." You know, using and stuff like that really fucked me up. Sometimes I just had a gut feeling about people that would tell me, you know, how they'd react under certain situations, under certain kinds of pressure, and whether or not they'd know what to do to save their own ass. I just knew this was bad news with this dude.

I was gettin' real skinny, you know, my hair was real long, I was lookin' like shit. I was just gettin' kind of tired of things, and I kept runnin' out of money, and somehow the hits weren't getting as big any more because we were running out of houses, 'cause we weren't the only people who were robbing houses. There's some houses we'd go into and there'd be nothing in there of any value, and that would mean we'd have to work twice as hard and go to more houses and be twice as careful. So things, you know, weren't always working out as planned. I decided maybe I needed some help.

I ended up meetin' this guy named Larry, and he introduced me to AA [Alcoholics Anonymous], and he took me and I stayed in for about three months. Then I got an apartment with this guy named Doug, and we had this other guy named Jeff move in who was a chronic junkie. He was dealin' cocaine out of the apartment while I was trying to stay sober. Doug was dealin' acid out of the apartment, and I was just going to meetings all the time, and somehow things didn't work out and I didn't have a sponsor and everything else, and I wasn't attending as many meetings anymore or anything else. My program was real shaky.

My parents were givin' Larry like a thousand dollars a week to make sure I stayed clean and sober, and they bought me a car and all kinds of stuff. So finally I went back out and started using after this 'cause my program was real weak. And I went out shooting coke 'cause Jeff was in the apartment and he ended up gettin' a quarter ounce of cocaine and we did it, just straight out did all of it, you know, in one night, between three people, and I said, "Oh, you know, that wasn't so bad, it didn't kill me." And so at this point in time I was gettin' kinda lazy. I wasn't robbin' that many houses anymore and I started to go on a check-cashing spree. Somebody had brought up the idea to me and said, "Well, your parents, what are they gonna do, throw you in jail again? That didn't do any good last time. Fuck it, they'll probably just give up and just pay the shit."

And so I went out and cashed all kinds of checks, and finally during the end of my check-cashing binge I met a new guy by the name of Rich, who's now my best friend. I turned him on to shooting coke on his eighteenth birthday. And I hadn't quite turned eighteen yet, I was gonna turn eighteen in a few days. About two months after I turned eighteen, I'd cashed this check on my parents' account for close to about nine hundred bucks and gotten, you know, what was it, I think it was close to about fourteen grams of pure cocaine. You know, just excellent blow. I mean, it cloroxed when I was mixin' it up in the spoon; you could smell it, I mean the whole bit, the coke was clean, melted crystal clear in water, I mean, it was just primo. So we ended up in this guy's apartment and we started shootin' all the coke.

By this time, you know, we were just into shootin' the coke for a while and just not too mixed up in heroin. And I remember, I was gettin so delirious from doing so much cocaine—we had finished about half of that within about three hours between the two of us—I was beginning to shake and stuff. And I finally mixed up a shot where the taste came on—when you shoot cocaine you get a taste, it's like a vapor taste, you can taste it in your mouth, you can smell it, it's just real wild—and I could tell, since I'd been shooting up for so long, I could tell by the way the taste came on that I'd done too much. And my knees buckled and I ended up grabbin' onto this faucet to hold myself up, you know, and got a dead grip on the faucet, and I was coughin' up white foam, and I went completely under, just standing up, went completely under, just overdosed standing up.

I ended up throwin' up a few times and got real sick, you know, and I finally said, after I came down, "Rich, man, you know, that was fuckin' wild. You gotta try it." Then I proceeded to overdose my best friend. I thought it was, yeah, I thought the high was basically pretty wild. If I would've known I was gonna overdose him, I musta been pretty delirious at the time. So it was like I really, yeah, I was real fuckin' out of it, so it was like I really wasn't thinking. I mean anything that wasn't sobriety was wild, yeah. And it was like, I ended up, you know, givin' him this shot, and he went into convulsions and ended up pissin' in his pants and just—he had a nasty time, and after that it scared him so bad he never did it again. He just quit altogether.

I kept shootin' coke and heroin—I started up on the heroin again. And I started robbin' houses again. One morning right after, I get this call from this detective and he's basically telling me, "Yeah, Al, I've got you on some long-time burglaries, this that and the other, and you're history." The thing is, he was usin' scare tactics on me until he could get my old partner to talk, the guy I'd had that gut feeling about before, the guy who'd never robbed houses. He did it 'cause he needed the money, quote-unquote. This detective basically told me that he rat-finked on me. He spilled the beans in a big kinda way, and that I was gonna be goin' to jail for a long time now. I don't know why he called me on the phone. So I casually, you know, packed myself up, grabbed my money, threw on my clothes, and split out the back door.

They nailed me a couple streets away. A few black and whites pulled up and a few undercover cars, and some plainclothes came runnin' up, and I had a gun sticking out of my belt, and they said, "Very neatly pull the gun out and set it down." I did that and the whole bit and got all fucked over, and anyway, you know, from there I ended up goin' to County Jail, and I sat in there for about six, seven months. I fuckin' ended up goin' through some fuckin' nasty withdrawals. Achy joints and fuckin' sick to my stomach and the runs and the whole fuckin' bit, man. And the hot and the cold spells. I fuckin' couldn't stand it, man.

It was like, you know, I was finally tired. I was finally

sick and tired of being sick and tired. You know, I was through robbin' houses. I was just so sick of gettin' high, I just said fuck it, I didn't even try to score in the can. After that, after the whole ordeal with the jail scene and being transferred from jail to jail, the judge finally put a sentence on me to go to the state pen for a year. So I sat in there for a year and finally got that all done. I came out in what was it, eight months and twenty days. All I did when I was in there was just pump iron and get mad, and think about how I was gonna kill this fuckhead who narked me off, basically.

When he was released from the state penitentiary, Allen entered a drug-rehabilitation program as mandated by the court. It was while in this program, his mind and body clear of drugs for almost a year now, that he began exploring his actions and their motivations.

I started to work in recovery and to learn why I did a lot of the things that I did. Basically, one reason I found out that I used drugs was acceptance: I never really felt a part of—like, even when I was in sixth grade, I never felt a part of the class. I never really had any friends, you know, and so drugs gave me that fulfilled feeling of "I can do anything the fuck I want and fuck everybody else's opinion of me." I ended up just learning a lot of stuff about myself and started to learn a lot about recovery and started to help other people, you know, really begin to enjoy—to help with people who were newer than I was. Being able to tell them, "Hey, you know, this is what works for me, maybe it can help you," and just passing on the message.

When I used, it just seemed like more or less something to do. Basically what I learned was I'm sick of payin' prices. I got sick of goin' to all these schools and sittin' in the jails and sittin' in all these places. I just got tired of it. You know, I realized it was my responsibility and not my parents' fault 'cause my parents, you know, my parents weren't the ones who were stickin' the drugs in my arms. I was the one who was stickin' all the drugs in my arms, and it's like I realized for myself that, you know what, it's my responsibility to quit doin' 'em. I started using out of curiosity, and then it no longer became curiosity, it became more or less to cover up the feelings. I wanted to cover up the way I felt about things, to make me so I could, you know, be more outstanding and go and talk with people that I normally wouldn't talk to. And it more or less made me a lot more crazy. I used to like to get drunk and go out and pick fights all the time. That was great for me.

I never thought I could do anything when I was sober. It's like, "What fun do these assholes have when they're sober?" You know, fuckin' normie, you know, normie fuckin' sober people—all they do is they act the same. And to me, it was like they're all just clones of each other, like it seemed they had the most dull and fuckin' boring life. I mean, all these fuckin' people are so plastic you can almost see the mold marks splitting around them. It just didn't seem, you know, realistic to me, you know, to hop up every morning and kiss your wife good-bye as you head to the job and hop in your car, you know, running out of your house with the white picket fence. That made me fuckin' ill. I said I wanted something different for myself. Yeah, I guess I definitely got something different, to say the least.

Now it's kinda like I look—I kinda look at the idea of the house with the white picket fence and everything else and, since I've seen the worst of things, it's like the worst that happens to me now sober is better than my best day using. It's like, nothing can happen to me today that really even stuns me that much. After seein' a lot of shit that I saw, you know, and goin' through what I went through, nothing's that big of a deal these days.

If somebody would've told me when I was goin' around snatching those drinks from my folks' table that I'd get to this point, I would've probably told 'em to get the fuck out of my face. No way that would happen to me. It's like I remember in sixth grade, seeing these movies like: "See Betty, see Betty take pills," and it shows this lady takin' these pills, and: "See Betty now, and her car's wrapped around a pole," and I used to always bust up at that shit. I said that'll never be me. You know, it'll never, it'll never happen to me. I finally realized, when I was about seventeen, that I was like Betty. It took me a long time to realize that. It was like I was in total denial. I wouldn't admit that, you know, Allen's a junkie. I wasn't willing to admit it.

I finally came to the reality of it later on. I was finally able to say, "I am, you know, I am a fuckin' junkie." And after a while it just got so I could admit it. I've been sober nine and a half months now, and things are goin' well. I'm living, I'm clean. Things are a lot better. It's like, after goin' through all the jails and shit—I mean, a lot of people don't really understand how much freedom they do have out here; until you've had all your freedom taken from you, every last bit of it—to where somebody's tellin' you when to shit, walk, talk, and eat, man—you don't know. And dope does that to you. That's how you end up. It's not a pleasant feeling. Especially being locked up like a fuckin' animal. And it gets real tiring. Things just finally got old and stale. I just got sick of the way I was living life.

There's nothin', there's nothin' I can really tell anyone, you know, if somebody's using, just maybe where I came from, you know, and what's happened to me, and that what I went through was just pure fuckin' hell. You know, shootin' dope and comin' down all the time and tryin' to scrape for my next fix and ending up in the jails, and listening to people getting beaten up all the time and listening about people gettin' raped and the whole bit—it's not real pleasant. It's not real pleasant at all. All the shit that I went through, you know, it's just horrible. And if people who are using now could just see what's actually happening, just actually believe it—you know, a lot of people say, "Ah, nah, I'll never end up in the penitentiary. I'll never end up, you know, gettin' hooked on this that and the other." But once it happens, and it's got you in its motherfuckin' grip, there ain't nothin' you can do, 'cause then it's all about ball and chain. You're hooked to it and it's hooked to you.

# JOHN

**"I've been to hell and back. The thing was, at the time, I thought I was in heaven."**

I was twelve when a bunch of my friends and I decided to just smoke some pot. We were real curious about it because we'd heard all about it, a lot from their older brothers and sisters. I'd always thought, "Oh my God, I'll never use drugs." My parents had gotten divorced the year before, and I thought, "Well shit, nothing's going right, so I'll just do it." It was so goddamned scary the first time, but it made me feel great. I loved it. I was shakin' right before we lit up, 'cause I'd always thought I'd never do drugs, which was a real laugh considering my father is a pharmacist. After that I really didn't think about doing any other drugs—I'd found the wonder drug. Pot was my best friend for a while, that's for sure. It was always there when I needed it. It eventually got to the point where I wouldn't go anywhere without it.

The man who lived next to me was a county coroner, and he grew the most amazing, powerful pot you've ever seen. I was friends with his son, and we used to go over there after school and steal a few buds out of the freezer, which was where he kept his stash. I mean, this was butt-kicking shit. What happened was, one day he caught us red-handed in the freezer. He got real pissed about it, not 'cause we were stealing, but because we were smoking. I couldn't believe that. Here was this guy, a pathologist, getting stoned, growing his own pot, and he's pissed at us. It was bullshit. It was hypocrisy. Anyway, he told my mom, who kicked me out of the house. She went bananas. That was more bullshit. She was a real fucked-up lady. She was an asshole. She used to hit me a lot. She drank all the time, plus she took a lot of Valiums and other stuff like that. I used to think, "You know, I don't drink, I smoke pot." Maybe she was pissed off at the world 'cause she and my dad had just gotten a divorce. But she was like that before, anyway. I think she had a bad childhood. Pretty much my dad couldn't take it anymore, which is why they got divorced. I was glad she kicked me out. She was always ragging on me. Nothing I did ever pleased her or satisfied her. I may not have been perfect, but at least I wasn't takin' all my anger out on everyone around me. I used to get all A's, but she was always pissed that I wasn't getting A-pluses. What a bitch.

**John, nineteen, came from a wealthy family. An only child, he was thirteen when his mother sent him to live with his father, who owned a chain of drugstores.**

Obviously, my dad knew I smoked pot, but he said he didn't care about it as long as I just didn't make it a problem—you know, it didn't hurt me in my grades in school or anything. So it was no big deal. He was real cool. He used to write notes for me in school so that I could take off and go surfing with my friends. Once, when I was fifteen, we went down to Mexico together and got stoned together. I was staying with him in his condo, but he was hardly ever there anyway, he stayed most of the time at his girlfriend's place. It was great. My friends and I could party as much as we wanted.

I never drank anything, 'cause I have a bad stomach. And I was really scared of pills and stuff like that. So I just smoked pot, and I smoked a lot of it. Everyday, a few times a day—before school, after school, sometimes I'd sneak out the back, through a window, or out at lunchtime, and come back all high. And I kept my grades up, all A's, so my dad didn't care. 'Course, he didn't know, I'm sure, how much I was smoking. I didn't want to do anything else, other than pot, but I got sick of it after a couple of years. I needed something to spice up my highs.

What happened was, my cousins had a lot of coke, and I was staying with my cousins for a while, and they were doing it, so I tried it. I liked it a lot—do a few lines, take a couple hits off a bong. It felt great. I got it for free from them, but then my cousin who had it left to go back to Colorado, so I just got an ounce from him and started selling it. What happened was, I stole a jar of Quaaludes from my dad's drugstore, where I worked after school, and I traded them for the coke. I stole a thousand 714s. I kept about twenty of 'em and took one just to see, but like I said, I was scared of pills. I gave the rest to a friend of mine, who kind of OD'd on them. He didn't die, but he went into a coma for a while.

So anyway, I started dealing the coke, scraping some off for me and my friends and dealing the rest. I was making a ton of money, stashing it in a safe-deposit box, and we were doing it just basically on the weekends. That's how it was for a long time, and then I started doing it just about every day. My dad was spending a lot of time at his girlfriend's house, and I had the condo all to myself, and my friends would come over and we'd snort and freebase. It turned into an everyday thing about then. I wasn't worried about getting addicted or shit like that, 'cause I'd always heard that coke couldn't be addicting. That's what they always said, that's what I always heard. I thought it was no big deal, 'cause I didn't do it all day long—I'd wait till nighttime, you know. It was there and fun.

That's when I started stealing Valiums and a couple other downers from my dad's stores, just to come down at night and go to sleep. They were going through them at the pharmacy like candy anyway, so I'd just take some out of the jar and they wouldn't ever know. Like, if there was a bottle of a thousand, I'd take about a hundred and fifty, or I'd hit it a few times, like fifty or sixty at a time. I was giving 'em to my friends too, so we could all calm down, so they'd last about a week or so. I think I was addicted to Valiums too. I was eatin' 'em all the time, waking up in the middle of the night. It's weird, 'cause I thought I wasn't addicted to coke 'cause I had the Valiums, which calmed me down enough to go to sleep at night so I wouldn't be up and watch the sun rise 'cause of the coke. But I was addicted to both.

I stopped taking Valiums when my dad caught me stealin 'em, so I had to stop working at the drugstore. That's when I started taking heroin a bit, just to calm down. I bought it from another kid I knew. I didn't shoot it, just snorted it, but I cut it out after a week or so. I thought, "Oh, my God, I'm a heroin addict or something." Actually, that's when I knew I was doing too many drugs and stuff. But I couldn't stop, 'cause they were always around, you know, wherever I went. All my friends had them.

Before that, though, I copped some amazing pharmaceutical coke from my dad's stores. They had it there for people with throat cancer. These couple of old ladies had throat cancer and they'd mix it up with morphine. One day, you know, he went in the back and I went and snagged it, went into the little safe part where they had it and took about a half ounce. That shit was pure. They keep it in a poison bottle, one that has a skull and crossbones on it. Any time you see that you know it's good shit.

It was like, at that point, I really didn't care whether I lived or died. I was always tryin' to do as much as I could, you know, get higher and higher. Nothing was goin' right, everything was fucked. I didn't care about anything. My dad was never around. At the time I thought he was cool, you know, giving me notes to ditch school, letting me run wild in his condo, getting high with me, but I don't know if I'd do the same for my son. At least, not as much as he did. I knew he cared about me, but he just didn't spend any time with me. He didn't know how, really, to make me happy. He'd give me money, you know, and everything I wanted, but we never did anything together or anything. The time he wasn't working, he'd spend with girlfriends or sitting in front of the television, jellin' out.

I had a lot of friends, but it was all just 'cause of drugs. I was pretty lonely. I didn't really relate with people at school. Everyone was all bopped out, you know. They were just all really into themselves, real selfish people, real gaudy, you know, rich kids—had to wear Guess clothes, and the girls dressed like Madonna and shit. Real trendy stuff. I just couldn't relate to anything except drugs. I had girlfriends, 'cause I had what they wanted: money and drugs.

It was great being stoned. It was, you know, it was great. I just could evade all the bullshit and just be stoned, do anything stoned—turn off the feelings. I just wanted to block everything out, is basically what it was. I don't know. I guess that's why I got as low as I did and my friends didn't: they could handle their feelings better than I could. When I wasn't high, I just wished I was. I guess I didn't feel good then. What I didn't know till lately was that I really didn't feel good when I was high—I didn't feel anything. After all I've been through, in some ways I definitely feel older than just nineteen, older than the other kids my age. But in some ways, definitely, I'm pretty immature now. Sort of I feel like I got robbed of my childhood. I do, I feel I robbed myself, you know, I paid the penalty. I mean, I don't remember a lot of what happened those years. It's just kind of blank.

**One thing John does remember is dealing drugs to support his habit.**

One of the guys I grew up with was the son of a Peruvian diplomat. He'd bring back incredible quantities of coke with him whenever he'd go back home for a while. I'm not sure whether his father knew or not what he was doing. Anyway, I was the middle man in a lot of deals, scraping a couple extra thousand off the top for getting someone a quarter pound of coke. Sometimes I'd buy some for myself too with the money I made scraping, and then I'd keep whatever I needed and sell when I needed money to buy more coke. I did a lot of wheeling and dealing. And it just fucked me up.

I was making so much money—as much or more than my father some months, sometimes $20,000 a month—that I moved out of my dad's condo when I was seventeen and rented this nice little house by myself. People came over all the time to get coke. There was so much late-night traffic and shit, people comin' by at two or three in the morning. I never slept hardly, and I was stoned all the time. When I wasn't stoned on coke, I'd be smokin' pot or takin' pills or shit. Man, I was really fucked up. I was snorting about three grams every night. The only thing I could think about was getting it or doing it, and then when I did it, it wasn't ever good enough. I never got high enough. It never really felt good.

One time, when I was a senior in high school, I fell off my motorcycle when I was stoned and broke my leg. I guess I'm lucky I didn't die, but I was so relaxed, I guess, when I hit that only my leg broke. Anyway, they gave me codeine for the pain, which was great, and I was out at my car freebasing before class. So I got in there, all stoned and everything, and I was supposed to be allowed to leave five minutes early because of my leg, but this bitch teacher always had it in for me. I guess I mouthed off at her a lot, though. You know, I didn't like school, all the pressure and everything. I was in advanced classes, you know, and I thought a lot of it was just bullshit, a waste of time. I thought I was beating the system. I went in there all stoned and happy and I thought that, you know, it was fun. But I didn't want to be there. Anyway, this time she wouldn't give me a pass to my counselor. I was twiddling my keys around my finger, and they fell off, and she picked them up and I asked her to give them back. But she wouldn't, she wouldn't give my keys back. I said, "May I please have my keys back." And she said, "No." And I said, "Listen, if you don't give me my keys back, I'll send someone back to get them." Well, I guess she took that as a threat on her life. They put me, right then, in this thirty-day drug program for threatening a state employee. That was fucked. As soon as I got out of there, I got high. It was just bullshit punishment to me.

Somehow, he says, John managed to graduate high school. But rather than enrolling in a four-year university, he began taking classes at a nearby junior college.

I was still stoned all the time, but I don't think anyone in my family knew. Anyway, my dad didn't. I guess he didn't know much of anything I was doing, 'cause he never asked me where I got the money to live the way I did. In fact, he used to give me money every month. He was probably glad I wasn't living in his place anymore. That way he didn't feel like he had to have the responsibility. I still have thirty-five thousand dollars in cash in a safe-deposit box in the bank. Anyway, I started going to this shitty little junior college near my house 'cause I didn't think I could be stoned all the time and go to the big university. My whole life I wanted to be a lawyer, but I lost a lot of ambition and a lot of energy. All I wanted to do was sit around and get stoned and kick back and do nothing. I don't know, I guess it was more fun. It felt better to be high and lazy than to work hard and deal with all the feelings and bullshit.

I started doing some more heroin too, 'cause nothing seemed to get me off the way I wanted. Then more Valiums. I was a real fucking wreck. About two thousand bucks a week was going up my nose, into my lungs, or in my arm. I couldn't even think straight. My Peruvian connection dried up, so I had to start dealing it kind of straight, so to speak. I started buying it from this guy I met who got it from this other guy who lived near the Mexican border. It was kind of scary stuff, but I didn't even think twice about it. One time we drove down there, to this house, and we were there for about fifteen minutes, and we were freebasing. My connection had just dropped off a kilo of coke. I was basically along for the ride, but what happened was, someone broke into this house where we were and tied everyone up. A girl who was there got shot in the neck and killed, and the guy we dropped it off to got shot in the shoulder. This other guy and I were left tied up in the house. When the police got there, they put us up on charges for dealing, but the charges were dropped almost right away 'cause the guy admitted it was his coke.

That really shook me up. I was just relying on drugs. Drugs were running my life, and this was the first time, if you can believe that, I could see that. So I decided to quit all the pills and heroin. And that was hell, sweating and dry heaves and shaking and fever. I just stayed at home and did it on my own. It took a month. No Valium, no heroin, no barbiturates. But when I finished, I wanted coke and pot more than ever. I couldn't wait, if I was out somewhere, to get where I could do a line or smoke a joint. Some nights, when my friends were over, I'd do seven grams of coke in the pipe. I got really crazy. I started leaving my doors and windows open, waiting for someone to try and come rob me, but I had a .357 Magnum this other guy had given me out on the table, and I was gonna blow their heads off, whoever they were. It didn't matter who—I just felt like someone was gonna come in sooner or later.

I was just hating life. I stayed at home the whole time. I wasn't eating or anything. Some of my friends would stop by. I just didn't have the energy to move. I kept waiting to die. It would have alleviated all the pain forever, but I didn't try to kill myself—not consciously. I guess I was doing a pretty good job of it, though. Nothing was fun anymore. I was paranoid and nervous all the time.

That was the low point for me. I don't know why, but I just kind of looked in the mirror one day and couldn't believe what I saw. It was like a ghost looking back. I found out later I'd lost fifty-five pounds. That's when I decided to stop everything. That was a fucking amazing experience. It was wild. I had hallucinations, weird things coming at me. After two weeks of that, I could tell I was getting better. But then I heard that a buddy of mine was sent to jail for fifteen years for dealing, and I thought, "Shit, everyone else is doing it, it won't kill me, I'll just do one gram." And one gram led to two, to five, to ten, and I ended up stayin' up for a whole weekend. What scared the shit out of me, what happened was, I started having seizures. I'd do some coke, and my whole body would start shaking. I'd just be on the ground, flailing around like a Cuisinart or something. Finally I called my aunt and told her I needed help. I didn't call my dad 'cause he had already told me a long time ago that quitting was just a matter of willpower, that you either do it or you don't. He thought I was just smokin' pot, maybe drinking a little, even after all that time. Actually, I guess, he probably knew what I was doing but I don't think he had the guts to approach me on it.

John's aunt placed him in an aggressive recovery center, where he had been for four months when interviewed. As the haze began to dissipate and he was able to think clearly for the first time in years, John began to put events into perspective.

I've got a hole in my sinuses from snorting cocaine. But that's good in a way, it'll keep reminding me, if I need any reminders. I've been to hell and back. The thing was, at the time I thought I was in heaven. I thought everything was great, but it just catches up to you—and it catches up quick. My world fell apart in a matter of weeks. I fucked myself up pretty good, I guess. Drugs ran my life. I couldn't wait to get high, get happy. But the thing is, I wasn't really happy. All that shit just got confused. When I wasn't high, I wished I was, and when I got high, I thought that's what feeling great was. But it wasn't. I wasn't feeling anything. That's why I took drugs—not to feel anything. Now I know what feeling great is, and that's how I want to stay.

# SUSAN

**"You think: What a waste, I've wasted my life. It'd be like a puzzle. If you took out all the times that I used or drank, there'd only be a few pieces left that were good. It'd be like a jigsaw puzzle with most of the pieces missing."**

I tried to commit suicide. I was just losing my mind. All I wanted was drugs and alcohol. All I wanted was cocaine. It was taking over my mind. I wasn't the same person any more. The shit really—it fucked me up.

Susan, twenty-one, is originally from a small town. Adopted by a lower-income couple after six years in foster care, she had two older brothers and one younger brother. She traces her drug use to the feelings caused by her father, who first tried to molest her when she was thirteen.

My father told me not to tell anybody. The only way he could try to do it was to try and get me drunk. He had a little brewery in the backyard, in the garage, where he'd make his own beer and wine, and he'd let me taste it all the time. I was about twelve or thirteen, right when I got into junior high, and he let me taste a little too much, and sometimes I'd just, I'd get so drunk or I'd get tipsy, and I'd get feelin' good. And I just remember a lot of the things he did. He tried to get one of my friends to go along with it, to get me and my friend at the same time. What a bastard he was.

He told me not to tell. He said he'd deny it. I just knew that—that there was something wrong, you know, the things that he was trying to do to me. He wanted me to watch him and my mom have sex. If my mother had known what he was saying, she would have—I don't know. That's why I was always so afraid to say anything, 'cause I didn't want my mother to be hurt. And I never knew when I was younger that she'd deny it, and so . . . I didn't have the guts to tell her when I was sober. So I had to get drunk, and then I finally got so angry and so pissed off at my dad I had to, I had to tell her once and for all because I knew I was leaving that night, and I knew I wasn't gonna ever be back. I was just gonna move out, get the hell out of there.

Susan mixed rubbing alcohol and orange juice—"a rough screwdriver," she called it—with several tranquilizers and a lot of cocaine in order to gather the courage to tell her mother about her father's actions. Just a few days before, her father had waited for her in her bedroom, naked, a bottle of grain alcohol between his legs.

I was on too much shit to get sick from mixing it all. The alcohol didn't bother me. It didn't really affect me. I just wanted some alcohol. Anyway, when I was all fucked up on that shit I told my mother about it, what my father did. I told her for the first time. And she fuckin' didn't believe me. She didn't fuckin' believe me. She told me I was a liar and all. And that's when I went up to the park. I was really fucked up. So loaded still from all the shit. I was just wasted. You know, it was all, it's still just kind of fuzzy to me, and all that shit that night, but I remember sitting under the tree, at the park, and I was just, I had nothing. I felt I had hit rock bottom. I'd completely lost my family, because I have—I had left so many times, I—I went up to the park and I had a razor blade and I just started slashing myself. The blade was dull, you know, but I cut pretty deep here on my wrist. And I had cut my face up before. I got scars.

**Susan has been trying, in therapy, to deal with the origins of her suicidal feelings, which are exacerbated by her drug use.**

There was a couple times I'd, you know, I'd try—I'd cut myself up just so I could get attention from my parents. I've tried to OD several times, on codeine, and aspirin, and anything I can get my hands on. I've used a knife, blades, beer cans, beer bottles, anything. The first time I did it, I think I was fifteen. I wasn't getting the attention, really, from my mother; it was always my little brother, it was always John somehow. It's kind of silly, now that I think about it, but she babied him, and my two older brothers, you know, they were in the military for the longest time, and I felt like an outcast, so I, you know, I would just . . .

It wasn't like that when I was a kid, before my father got weird on me. I had a lot of friends. I was just gettin' out of the Barbie doll stage at that time, when my father first tried, you know. I had a lot of close friends that I continued to keep till I graduated from high school. So I always had the same friends, and then we all did our drugs together. We all used together. And most of my friends knew what the hell my dad was doing to me. They knew. But they weren't gonna say anything. They were there for me, you know, they helped me out a lot.

I graduated from high school, and I went in the Army right after that. I joined the Army because I was psychologically . . . Deep down inside I didn't want to go out and look for a job, and I was living with my brother and his wife at the time because I wasn't getting along with my parents, and we were using, and I was pushing drugs at school for my brother, you know, dealing for my brother at school. And I was getting drunk every night. And eventually I knew that I was scared to death because I wasn't gonna have any more school; all my friends weren't gonna be there, I wasn't gonna have any place to go when school ended. Yeah, things weren't goin' right. I guess you could say that. It was either get a job or babysit the whole summer, and I didn't want to babysit, so I decided I was gonna do something, maybe just try to get off the drugs and alcohol. And do something. So I went in and I became an administrative specialist. And I made it through basic training, and got halfway through AIT [Advanced Individual Training]. During basic training you couldn't do any drugs, and it felt good, although they had a lot of physical strain on me—you know, you were constantly doing something physical.

I mean, but I couldn't wait for that beer at the end of the six weeks. So the first day I got out of basic training I went out and got drunk, and I passed out. My buddies caught me and they had to carry me back and I got sent to the company commander and all that shit, you know, and I really got busted. Because I made an ass of myself. That didn't bother me, though. I continued to drink and they'd smuggle some weed in, and some cocaine, and we'd have a little party up in the barracks.

Oh God, you know, we had these little fans up in the ceiling of the barracks that blew out the marijuana smoke, and we'd be in there smokin' and talkin' and it was late at night, and we were always bummed out 'cause we had to get up at four-thirty every morning. Every morning, you know, we all felt like shit. We always went to bed stoned, even though we knew we'd have to get up early. I woke up stoned, you know. I was doing a lot of cocaine, and I'd usually get about two to three hours' sleep and that'd be enough. I'd sometimes get up and have a toot in the morning, and that'd get me going.

I was all fucked up in the class one day and I just went up and told my sergeant that I didn't wanna be in the Army anymore, and that I'd been using and I just—I couldn't take it, 'cause I was, I mean, I was just a wreck. That's how I got out, on a medical discharge. And, you know, I'd tried suicide when I was in the Army too, you know. And they didn't find out about it 'cause it was in the winter and my arms were all fucked up, and I got to cover it up.

When I had it, I'd snort coke all day. Even when I got out, I'd got to the point where I was begging my friends to go get me some. I had the money, and we'd drive all over town, all day long, just tryin' to get a gram, and . . . I was a waitress for the longest time, and I'd do coke to get my tips, 'cause when I'd do cocaine, I was a good waitress. I was able to be on the ball and do things just like that. And I made some good money on tips. And also, I kept puttin' money in the bank and saving it, and then I'd get on these drunks where I'd just take my money out of the bank and split. Bus, plane, train, car, whatever. I usually liked to take a bus because I liked to sit in the back of the bus and get loaded and watch the country go by. That felt, I don't know, that felt safe.

I'd just work and save up enough money and then split. I've ended up in Texas on drunks, I've ended up in Georgia, Kentucky . . . Getting there felt good, and then once I'd get there I was scared to death all over again. I'd done so much shit, I had a warrant out for my arrest in Texas. I don't even know what I did. I'm too afraid to ask. My mom and dad know about it. They don't even know what I did. All I know was that I was drunk the whole two weeks I was there. I was living with my brother's friend. We were supposed to get married. That sounds weird, huh? Yeah, I was supposed to get married, and—I just got scared. I didn't wanna get married, and so I drank. I tried to tell him that I don't wanna get married, and I want to go back home. I'd known him all my life, you know. I've known him all my life. He was always around, always . . . And then he moved out of state, moved near my brother. He wasn't an alcoholic, he just, he didn't know me very well. I was a drunk. I didn't know whether to try, but . . . He lived in a bachelor apartment, and there were guys all over, a swimming pool, jacuzzi—everything. And he bought me all the beer I wanted. And he'd go to work and I'd have the whole place to myself. And I'd just get buzzed every day, all day long. And I'd end up with somebody. One of the guys in the apartment building, you know, I'd end up with one of them. They always . . . And that's when I felt real . . . And then I split. I borrowed the money from one of the guys and I hopped on a plane and went back home. I really did a lot of traveling. In the past three years I've done the most traveling. And I don't know how I'm alive right now, because I did some very terrible and crazy things.

I really, I'm angry still. I've tried to kill my father a couple times. I put a lighter in his gas tank one time, but the car wouldn't start, so that backfired. And he's a diabetic, so one night, I got a—you know, I got a—I was insane, I was totally insane. I was all wired up on cocaine and shit. He has to eat at a certain time. It was supposed to be my job to feed him when my mom wasn't there. He told me not to worry about it, you know, 'cause I was always makin' sure he—I've always pretended that I loved him, and I really cared for him. "Oh, you better eat," I'd tell him. Shit like that. So here I am, and he fell asleep, and I didn't wake him up, and my mom was gone, out of town that weekend, it was just me and him, and so I sat in my bed all night long, you know, I sat up waitin' for him to die, and I heard my mom come home early in the morning. Shit, you know, she found my dad on the kitchen floor. He had insulin reactions, and if she didn't come home that morning my dad would've been dead. She wasn't supposed to come home that morning. He would have died, in the insulin reaction. And I—she just came in and I just pretended I was sleeping. And my whole body was shakin', you know, I was shakin' so bad. And I thought to myself, "My God, I really, I tried to kill somebody. I'm, you know, homicidal." I really was, you know, I really would've, if I had a gun, man, I would've blown his head off. I'd be in jail today as a murderer. I was all fucked up on the drugs. I couldn't even think straight. I didn't know up from down. Coke, downers, alcohol, anything I could take not to feel anything. I don't know, man, I don't think I was human, or anything like that, anymore.

It went on until—it really kind of stopped about three years ago. It stopped, 'cause that's when I split. He'd still give me the looks, the looks, and—he tried several times. And with my friends, too. He's a sick man. And then he turns around, you know, and calls me an alcoholic, and calls me this and that, and everything. He's a sick man, and I'm sick, but I'm getting better.

I just recently talked to my mother for the first time in three months, and it pisses me off, because she still pretends that there's nothing wrong. She pretends, she's just pretending that everything's all right. Great, I'm in a recovery home, and they know that I'm never gonna see 'em again, because I don't, I—I don't even think they want to see me anymore. I talked to her. I just told her in the end that I loved her, and she just said good-bye and hung up.

After three months of detox, rehabilitation, and therapy, Susan has just begun to find herself again—to find the person who had survived beneath the unrelenting torpor brought on by drugs and alcohol. It has been a difficult process, sorting through the memories and experiences, trying to put them in order.

I smoked pot for the first time in eighth grade, when I was about fourteen. I began drinkin' a lot the year or so before. By the time I was sixteen I had to drink every day. I started on speed when I was fifteen. That's when I started pushin' it for my brother, and I sold it for him all through high school. That's how I had my friends, 'cause they knew that Susan had speed. Then, when I was sixteen, I went over to my rich cousin's house. I was drunk, and she took this stuff and started rubbing it on my gum, and I said, "What are you doing?" And she gave me some of this coke, and I was feeling pretty good, and I called her the next day and I told her, you know, thanks. And from then on, you know, I had to have cocaine and I had to score.

Right now, I mean, I wanna go out and—I mean I want a line so bad, you know, I can taste it. Right now. I know I'm not supposed to. I just want it, though. Coke. Yeah, and whiskey, just anything that'll make it so my head can't function, so I don't have to feel anything, 'cause I don't like to feel. You know, now I'm starting to feel. Now that I've been clean awhile, I'm starting to feel, and it really hurts. This, you know, they say it'll pass, it'll pass. Well, it's been three months and I'm just starting, you know, I've been really depressed. When you've been getting loaded every day just about for eight years, three months isn't very long. You don't get a chance to grow up. I think of all the times where I—where one time I really, I got scared. I was, I wanted to, I really wanted to kill myself. And I had taken a lot of pills and I started feeling, I started feeling it, you know: My heartbeat was getting really slow and hard and I started writing a suicide letter. And I still got that suicide note. I still have it. It's just all slurred language, you know, 'cause I couldn't see straight, I couldn't write. I said somethin' like, "I loved you, but please don't be angry at me." It was to my parents. And at the end, it—I remember the pen was running out of ink and I just scratched it in with the pen, and I said, "I've just been hurting all these fucking years," and it just—I let somebody read it and they freaked out. I still have it, and it's in a little book of mine that I . . . The only paper—I couldn't even get out of bed to get a piece of paper, so I had to grab a book and write it in the back of a book. And I still got that book.

I remember, I slept for three days. I thought I was dead. I thought I was dead. I ended up in the hospital. I woke up in the hospital. I couldn't figure out what was wrong. I was strapped down, my legs were strapped down, my arms were strapped down. They wouldn't let me out of there. They wouldn't even let me get up to go to the bathroom. I had to lay there for three fucking days. And they wouldn't come—nobody'd come see me. I felt like shit. They were gonna—they put me in the psych ward for one day, you know, because they just, they evaluated me. They told me I wasn't crazy, I wasn't nuts. You know, I thought I was.

I'm kind of grateful that he's not my real father. She's not my real mother. I was adopted when I was six years old. Before then I lived in foster homes and orphanages, you know. And I remember a lot of that too. I had gotten beat. I got beat 'cause they kept tellin' me to go over to the corner and say hello to a rubber plant. I remember that shit so clearly, and I kept sayin' hello to the rubber plant, and this man was beatin' me. I was about five years old. Right before I got adopted.

And they put me in a—my foster mother came home, and they put me in a tub of ice cubes. So I wouldn't bruise, you know, and I got really sick, and that's when they took me out. And that's when I was finally adopted.

To help her stay clean after she finishes rehab, Susan plans to go back into the Army—a place, she believes, that provides the discipline and structure she needs. She says she feels cheated out of her childhood, having realized early in life that there were many things she'd never be able to accomplish.

It seems funny now, but I remember I wanted to be an airline stewardess, I wanted to be a secretary, I wanted to be a mom. I think when I was six, I really wanted to be Barbie. I remember, yeah, I was—I wanted to be somebody famous. You know, one time, I thought, you know, it'd be nice if I could've been the President of the United States. And then when I was starting to get out of high school, I was seriously thinking about getting into airlines. To be a stewardess. But instead I went into the Army. I didn't have the patience, I didn't want to go through the schooling to be a stewardess. I'm very aggressive, you know, very aggressive, bullheaded. My mom and dad keep throwing that shit at me. And I don't know why. I've just been like that all my life. Stubborn, bull-headed, defensive. "Don't touch me, don't talk to me," you know, "don't tell me what to do." And I stop and look at the things that I . . . And I'm trying to change that but it's really hard because of all the stuff that I'm so used to doing all my life. It's not like flipping a record over to play a different song, you know. You can't do that. It's gonna take a lot more time.

I still, you know, I really want—I don't want to do drugs anymore. Or I should say, I can't. I still want to but I can't. I find myself, you know, wanting to pull my hair out of my head because I just don't think I can do it. I just want drugs. I wanta get high. I just keep wanting to get high. Anything.

I wanted to grow, and my parents were always pullin' me back. So I did drugs instead. They helped me escape from the feelings of being angry, feelings of bein' hurt, feelings of just flat out feeling sorry for myself. When I did drugs I had the ambition to do something, to feel like I was somebody. Yeah, 'cause I didn't have to, I wasn't myself, I didn't have to look at Susan. I didn't have to look at me. 'Cause I was disgusted with myself, I hated myself, I didn't feel good about myself. That's why other people didn't like me. I thought I was just a big mistake in life itself, for being here.

At the beginning, I thought I was pretty much in control of the drugs and I liked the way they made me feel, and then things started getting out of control. Until I started slashing my arms up, I just didn't realize what happened to me. It's like I was dreamin'. Because I didn't think like this when I was sober, I didn't have the guts to do it. You know, some other time I did it maybe just for attention. I still feel like a baby. If I had it to do all over again, I'd be open now. I would, I'd learn to be open now, to tell the truth, to say exactly how I feel. That's got to be so much better than taking drugs. Drugs just make you someone else, someone other than you are.

But I gotta say, in three months I, you know, I have learned to do that, to open up and tell people how I'm feeling. Some of the times I don't feel better when I tell people how I'm feeling. I, you know, I want to run across the street 'cause I'm twenty-one now and I can go and buy liquor now if I want. And that scares me, because when I was in the alcohol rehab for a thirty-day program, I turned twenty-one when I was in there and I wanted to leave on my birthday and go get drunk and celebrate 'cause I was twenty-one, and I thought to myself: My God, twenty-one years old now, and I can't drink anymore, I can't . . . And I started crying because I had used it all up before I was even legally able to do it, you know—to go party and have a good time, and. . . .

I don't go to them places anymore. But if I was gonna drink I'd go to a liquor store and just get a bottle. Sit wherever and just—I don't know. Even talking about it, I get all revved up inside. And it scares me because I really—sometimes I just want to say "Fuck it all" and go out and get drunk, and just go down and be on Skid Row and hit rock bottom. But I keep thinkin': "Well, you do that again, honey, and you ain't ever gonna make it back." Because they told me, I was told that if I ever was to drink again, I'd die. I'm not suicidal anymore, and I don't want to be like that.

I think of all my friends right now that I went to school with, and they're using still today. That's how I got like them, you know. I turned into them, because I was usually a shy, quiet person. And I wanted to be more like everyone else. I wanted to be like them. But I guess I'm not like them. They never—they never abused this shit like I did. I don't know why some people can and some can't. But you never know who you are. Anybody could do like that, like I did. Well, I'm one of the people who can't. I can't handle it.

I just look at myself and I can't believe the shit that I've done, the shit that I've been through. It doesn't seem possible. You know, I've never been in jail, but I've almost been beaten up by cops. You know, beat upside the head with clubs and shit when I was loaded. I've mouthed off to people. I become a completely different person when I'm loaded—I don't know who, just someone different—and that different person thinks she's got it under control, thinks she's right. I wanted to beat up an old man one night and they had to pull me off of him. I don't know what was said, but I remember that I almost got put in jail for assault. And that's not me when I'm sober. I get angry more now, though. I punched the wall a few weeks ago and had a dislocated knuckle because I wanted to hit one of the guys here. I just like to feel pain. When I feel pain when I'm angry, it relieves me, it relieves all that stress—all the emotional pain. And I feel better. I laugh after I do something like that.

I'd probably be working in an office, a big corporation or something by now. If I'd been able to stay away from drugs, even with my dad and all like that, I *would* have a good job today, and have a nice car, probably be married, you know. Maybe even have a baby, you know, 'cause I was supposed to get married when I was eighteen to another guy, and I knew, you know, the date was coming up, and this guy, he really wanted to get married, and he didn't drink or nothin'. And he was willing to, and I wasn't, 'cause I was drinking, and now today, I think: "God, why did I let him get away?" Why did I? That could have been it, right there, you know, and I could've had a nice job, I could've still been in the Army, had a good rank, good pay, without the drugs and the alcohol, you know. I know, I know I could've been somewhere today, instead of sittin' right here. I could have been somewhere out there, being somebody, you know, somebody different, instead of an addict and an alcoholic.

I only did heroin a couple times. I was scared. I guess I wasn't scared of the other drugs 'cause I'd been doing them for so long. I knew I was just . . . Cocaine was really right, 'cause it—I knew how it was gonna make me feel, and I knew what to mix it with. I based coke a lot too, you know, and I drank. I did everything. I took pills, I didn't even know what they were, just because they were there, and sometimes they didn't even do nothin' to me. I was just a junkie, I was all—I mean, I was sick. I was so sick, I'd be walking around campus in high school and I'd see a pill on the ground and I'd pick it up and pop it in my mouth, not even knowing what it was.

The first time she ever took a drink, Susan was eight. She wanted to please her older brother, who had given her a bottle of sweet wine while driving on a rural highway; she vomited several times, her head hanging out the window. Now she fears that her nephew, eight years old, will also become an alcoholic/addict because her brother gives him all the beer the boy wants.

My brother was a crazy motherfucker, he was. All three of my brothers were so different. And I had one brother who I used to deal for at school. He used to give me anything I wanted—beer, wine, anything—to deal for him. When I went in the Army, they threw me a big party and my mom even came, and we had a big keg of beer, and my brother gave me a dime bag of speed, and I did a lot of speed and I did a lot of whatever.

Everything but heroin. I just, I've seen what it can do, I've seen some of my friends freak out from that shit. And I just—I guess it was just fear of maybe my mom and dad finding out. I don't know. They knew about the cocaine, 'cause they found shit in my room, and they told me if they found it again that I was out and they would call the police. I just said, "Fuck it," and I just kept doin' it and they never—you know, I just kind of hid it between my mattress in my bedroom: my razor, my mirror, the straw.

My mom was stupid. My mom and dad are so blind. They've always threatened to kick me out, but I moved out more than they threatened. When I ran away, I didn't make contact with them. I never called 'em. I didn't write 'em. When I ended up in the South I didn't call 'em for like eight or nine months. I was doin' real good there. I had a good job, I was a supervisor. I was supervising a hamburger stand, and I'd really gotten the hang of that, and I was working two jobs, I had my own apartment, and—I was doing real good. But it was so good it scared me, and I quit, and then I dropped it all and ran. I guess 'cause I've had so many negative things in my life happen to me, that I might—any time a good thing's gonna happen I get scared. And I can't handle good things, I guess, 'cause I'm not used to them. I don't know how to accept 'em. So I called my mom and dad and I told them I was gonna come home. And I packed all my bags, and I took a Greyhound bus down to the airport. Waitin' for my flight, I kept walkin' towards where you go onto the plane, and I kept walking back to the door, the exit to get out of the airport. I kept walking back and forth, couldn't make up my mind. And I split. And I got back on the bus and came back, called the landlord and got my apartment back, got my job back and everything. You know, like, desperation.

Drinking heavily, Susan began calling in sick. She and her friend, Liz, had since met a wealthy fifty-eight-year-old woman whose severe back problems forced her to take strong medication for the pain. In need of full-time assistance, she invited the two girls to move in with her in exchange for minimal care. What she didn't know was that the girls were stealing her drugs.

All I had to do was stay there and take care of her. Take her pills, cook her dinner, and take her pills, and put her to bed, and take some more of her pills. She never noticed her pills were missing. She never knew it. I took everything she had. Ruby had everything, and I remember one time she couldn't drive and I had to drive her car for her. And I got in, and I was seeing three steering wheels. I was gonna get in it and drive that car, and it's like the whole front of the hood was just getting longer, and things were just being pushed away from me, and I knew I was hallucinating. I was hallucinating and I said, "I can't do this, I can't." I couldn't even hold on to the steering wheel because I didn't know which one I was holding on to. And it was one steering wheel, really. And I was seeing three. I remember that I said, "Ruby, don't make me drive. I can't drive."

There were just so many different pills, so many of 'em. I didn't care what they were. It was just, it was fun. It was so—oh, I loved it. I didn't have to feel anything. I didn't want to sit there and take care of an old woman all day long. I didn't wanna do that. Fuck. So I'd be able to take these pills and drink beer and she'd kind of get on my butt about drinkin'. She didn't have any idea I was taking her pills, and I'd be fucked up all day long and she wouldn't know it. I'd be flyin'. And me and Liz'd go out all night long and just drink until we couldn't drink no more, and just—I really, I get scared when I think about that time because I'd gotten into so much shit. I was in and out of detox so many times. I was in detox at least three times a month. Three times a month. And I'd leave on an AMA [*Against Medical Advice*]. And they'd give me this tranquilizer, Xanax. And this is another little trick I pulled when I was in detox so I'd get my, you know—I'd just pretend I was a nervous wreck and I needed something, so they'd give me Xanax. These little purple footballs. And they'd give me one, three or four times a day, to calm my nerves down. So I'd get one, and I'd pretend I was gonna take it, and I'd put it in my little pocket and then I'd have—like, I'd wait for two days and I'd have about six or seven of 'em, and I'd pop 'em all at one time. I'd be flyin', man. That shit was good.

Everywhere I went I always made sure I had somethin'. When I got back West, I found out my little brother was taking 'em. Xanax. And I got into them. And they just, they seemed to make the time go by so fast—just sit there and things would just start spinning and the arms on the clock'd just go round and round and round and round, and I'd feel happy. Susan's happy and Susan's somebody, you know, and I'd get drunk, and I'd go up to the grocery store, and I'd just get on the phone, and I'd just start calling anybody and talkin' to 'em on the telephone, and I wouldn't know who the hell I was talkin' to, but it was somebody.

See, when I'm not high, I'm still paranoid to go anywhere by myself. Even when I was living at home I'd . . . The store was right across the street from our house, and I was always scared to walk up there and get something, you know, if I needed a Coke or somethin'. But when I was drinking or when I was on somethin', man, get the hell out of my way, I'm goin', you know, I'm comin' up there, and I'd just hang around up there all day long, and I knew most of the people around there anyways and I'd still get scared.

My dad forced me to get a job I didn't want. I was working at a factory then. I always loved to do factory work because I could be wasted and they wouldn't know it. And my dad wanted me to get another job, and they had real good benefits. At the factory, I had to work for a certain amount of time, like three months, to get some benefits. And I was there my second month, and my dad made me quit and get a job at this restaurant I did not like. I didn't like it, I felt I was being pressured, so I quit. I got all coked up, and I—I worked there for about a month, and I quit, and they paid me right on the spot. And when my mom and dad asked where my money was, 'cause when I was living there they made me pay them, like, two hundred bucks a month, I told them I got fired and that they'd be giving me my check soon. I'd taken that money and I'd bought drugs and alcohol, over a hundred dollars I spent in one night. And on cocaine. I had this friend Amy, and we'd go out and buy cocaine and I'd stay out all night long. My mom and dad just got so used to me stayin' out all night long they wouldn't even ask me where I'd been—they wouldn't even say anything to me. Me and Amy, we used to always go in on a gram. My brother gave me money for selling his speed, so I had all this money and spent it on coke.

If I had a choice, I'd go out and buy cocaine and then I'd be able to get some booze after that. If someone gave me a hundred dollars right now, I'd want cocaine first, but I'd have to have alcohol. I don't know, I gotta have—I don't like coming off coke. I don't like coming down from it. It's, it's just, it's not a good feeling. I remember, I had to drink two pots of coffee one night because I didn't have any more cocaine, and I didn't want to feel like coming down, so I drank two pots of coffee just to keep me up enough till I could get to the liquor store and get some liquor. They keep you on a—it's like you're on a scale and you're scalin', goin' like this—you're just, you're not so drunk where you're fallin' down, and you're not so wired up where you're too wired on coke.

When I didn't have the cocaine, I'd really, I'd go on an alcohol binge for the longest time. I wouldn't buy any cocaine for a long time. I tried to get off of it several times before I graduated from high school. I'd just get it away from me and I'd go two days and I'd just—I could still feel that shit comin' down my throat. I still feel it.

I can't stand to see other people go out and do what I did when I was a kid. I can't, I can't stand it. I want to do everything in my power to make 'em stay away from that shit. I try to tell 'em what I went through with it. I feel for people now. I care. And that's somethin' new to me. I care about people and I care about myself. If I see somebody crying, and I don't know what they're crying about, I'll start crying too. I feel it. I feel tears, you know. And it's scary. I guess that's why I cry, 'cause it's—it's really scary having feelings. After three months' sobriety, it's just like being a baby again. You know, I'm living now, I'm learning, but I'm twenty-one. I'm not six years old. And I—it kind of makes me sick to my stomach, 'cause you kind of think: What a waste, I've wasted my life. I wasted a lot.

Just last night I was thinking to myself, you know, I keep getting these memories of when I was going to school, and the cloudy days, and how I'd go over to a friend's house. I remember Christmases; I hate thinking about Christmas because Christmas is always depressing for me because the family was all together and—I still think about the past. I keep looking back. It's really emotional for me to think about things like that because I just want to go back and do that shit all over again. Have the good, the good life I've had, the good times I've had with my family and my friends, and just leave out, leave out all the times that I used and drank. But then there wouldn't be much—there wouldn't be much in there. It'd be like a puzzle: If you took out all those pieces there'd only be a few pieces left that were, that were good. It's like a jigsaw puzzle with most of the pieces missing. You know, that's what I feel like my life is like.

# MICHAEL

**"The way I was feeling, it would've been okay if I died."**

When I was fifteen I was arrested by an undercover officer posing as a student in my high school. I swear, she didn't look older than sixteen. She asked me to sell her some pot, and when I did, she popped me. They let me off on probation because it was my first offense. I guess she popped a whole bunch of other people too, all about the same time. She was there three months. The funny thing is, when I got arrested for selling pot, I wasn't using it. Pot always made me feel burnt. I always got tired. I'd smoke it and sit on the corner and do nothing. I never really liked it, but I had to try it when my friends did; I didn't want to be left out. I sold it and didn't use, only 'cause I needed the money. I mean it wasn't my job, exactly, but my buddies and I usually went out to party on the weekends—you know, get some beer, a little coke, something else like acid—and I needed the money. It was a good way to make some extra bucks. Two dollars allowance a week doesn't really get you that much.

My main thing turned out to be alcohol. Alcohol was the best, 'cause it removed my inhibitions. I always felt inadequate to others. I was always shy, shy with girls and meeting people, and alcohol always made that a lot easier. That's why I eventually really stopped using everything else and just drank.

**Michael, nineteen, was adopted at birth by a couple who divorced only three years later. He was their only child.**

My mom didn't know till she got a phone call from the county telling her I'd been arrested that I was even using pot. She got real pissed off, and I was grounded for about two months. I think that was good on her part because that's what's really got me out of the pot scene. That really did a good turn for me because I was getting fails in school. I was ditching so much school that I couldn't go back, because I didn't have an excuse for all the days I'd ditched. And once I got arrested, it put me in a continuation, and from there on I was gettin' like four-point averages. I told her "Fuck you" a couple times, but basically I held to the grounding because if I was good for a week, I'd get the other week off, or, you know, she'd loosen it up a little bit. It was always hard for her to stick to her punishments.

She was pretty easygoing with my grades, like in high school and stuff. She didn't care just so long as I passed, she said, as long as I did my best. That was pretty nice. She was a little overprotective, though. She always wanted to know where I was going, and when I'd be back; she wanted the phone number of where I was going, and stuff like that. So I ended up giving her wrong numbers and stuff, you know, so she couldn't call this person's house, so if we were all wasted . . .

After my parents got divorced, I saw my dad only about once a month or so. We've never really gotten along very well. He's always expected more than what I could put out. Even when I put up a hundred percent. He's a lawyer and has his own law firm, and he always expected, you know, once I got out of high school with a four-point—which I was not able to keep up, there was just no way—that I'd do the same in college. But I couldn't do that either. Because by the time I got to college, I was gettin', like, three-point maximum, and that was like putting a hundred percent of my alcoholic mind into my work. But I always felt pressured that he wanted me to do better.

Michael said he was painfully shy as long as he could remember, with the only relief coming when he drank or snorted coke. "When I got buzzed," he said, "the shyness kind of disappeared. The shyness went away and the talkativeness came out."

Except for Valiums, I've never had a downer. I guess downs would have done the same thing as alcohol—you know, take away my inhibitions—but I didn't have the energy for them. You know, if I took a Valium I didn't have the energy to get up and start talkin' to people. And I never really did 'em all that much for that reason. I did 'em a couple times at my dad's house after he went to sleep. And I was by myself, and I was usually watching TV or something like that.

The first time I drank, I was six years old. It was at a family thing, and I guess they thought it was cute and gave me a little wine. Just a little. But I never really got drunk. I can't remember being drunk. The first time I ever really went out and specifically got drunk was probably when I met this girl. It was during the summer. I think I was, like, thirteen, and that was the first time. She was babysitting at this person's house, and we had screwdrivers. She was drinking 'em, not exactly like water, but she had a bunch. And I had like one, and that was enough for me. I don't remember exactly, but I probably did it because I liked her and I wanted to get laid: "Yeah, let's drink some screwdrivers." And it worked. I also got in trouble for it. But at that time, my doing it outweighed the consequences. You know, I would've done it again for the same type of punishment. You gotta measure the risks and the rewards, so if the reward is more than the risk . . . Anyway, after that, I had beers now and then. I can't remember exactly, you know, days or the exact experiences. But I didn't really drink that much at that time—a few beers here and there, basically—well, 'cause there was nothing else around, I think is what it was. Just to get buzzed. And just to escape reality for a little while. Probably if I'd had some pot around at the time, I'd have done that instead. At that time, you know, I think I was about fourteen and pot was the big thing.

I 'shroomed once in junior high school—in band class. I think I was about fourteen. My friend had some 'shrooms that came from Oregon, and he was sellin' 'em in the bathroom. He owed me ten bucks, so I said, "Just give me a gram and I'll do 'em right now." And he did, and I did 'em—right there in school. I almost got sent to the nurse, because I was just staring into space and at all the instruments and stuff. I played the drums, and the conductor asked me if I was feelin' okay, and I couldn't answer him 'cause it was like all warped and stuff, and I didn't answer him. After a while, I answered him and said I'll be okay. I was having heavy hallucinations, but it was only about an hour high, because after class I started mellowing out a little bit. That was the heavy pot-smoking year for me, so we—my friends and me—were getting stoned basically five days a week. It's a very psychological addiction, pot is, and so we were getting stoned on hash and pot in the mornings before school, then at lunchtime, out on the grass on the playing field. When I say five days, you know, that means out of the week—it might've been on the weekend, you know, depending on how the money situation was going. That's about when I started selling, 'cause I found a guy who had quantities. I could get a good deal for a certain amount, and then I'd pinch some out of the bag and that way I'd have pot and money. But like I said, it didn't take long after that till I got a little tired of smoking pot. I was more into beer. I didn't really know anything about coke then. I'd heard stories about it, but you know.

I should mention that I was also doing speed; black beauties was a big thing. And mini-whites, yeah. Oh, yeah, that was big all over school. I did 'em a lot of times. Once a week at least. I really don't know why exactly, 'cause it's hard to say, 'cause after a while it was just fun to do it, you know. We weren't having fun sober, we were not having fun whatsoever sober. It always seemed to be fun to get stoned together and laugh for no fuckin' reason at all—to sit around a room and just laugh. So that's basically why we all got stoned a lot.

I was gettin' plastered on the weekends, but not during school. I was trying to stay cool and get good grades. I found a liquor store where they would sell to me, they wouldn't card me. If there was no people around they wouldn't card you, 'cause my friends had done it. I mean, there was a guy that looked like he's twelve years old, and they'd sold to him before. I guess I drank mostly weekend parties and stuff, and it was great 'cause I hadn't seen my friends for a while after I put down on the drugs. Then my mom found out a couple times I was drinking. It wasn't a real big thing. I guess after the pot, which she'd freaked on, she took the beer pretty lightly. She rarely drinks. She'll have a little thing of amaretto, and she'll get a little buzz.

Oh yeah, I should say that I started doing a little coke about a couple months before I graduated—that's when it came into the scene. I went over to this girl Carol's house, and she had a party this weekend, and there was lots of coke goin' around. That was like, I think that was the first time I tried it—I'm not quite sure. Everybody was doing it. It was on a glass, on a mirror, and it was just goin' around the room. Yeah, it was just goin' around the room. And then I looked at it—what they were, you know, paying for this little bit, this little vial. It was a hundred bucks. Whoa! And this mirror's going around with mounds on it. I'm just going, "Whoa." Thousands of bucks worth of coke. God, yeah.

Drinking only moderately and still shying away, for the most part, from other drugs, Michael graduated from high school with pretty good grades when he was seventeen. At the same time, he and his other musician friends formed a band, which played several clubs around town. Michael's father, though, wanted to discourage him from pursuing his drumming career and offered to pay him $450 a month if he would study business law at a local junior college. Michael said yes to the deal and moved into his own apartment. He also found a job working part-time for the electric company, so between his father, the band's earnings, and his job, he had plenty of money to spend on alcohol.

I remember when I was like real young, asking my mom if we can get a drum set. I used to take coffee cans and take the plastic tops and use chopsticks on 'em, you know, like they were drums. I wanted to be a drummer all my life, but to my father you can't earn a living, you can't earn a decent living being a musician. All my dad listens to is elevator music. That's what he gets off on, and marching bands. I went to college for him. In a way, he was bribing me. "You go and study business law and I'll send you, you know, four hundred and a half a month." He was trying to get me out of music, he really was. And maybe, I don't know, maybe I was saying "Fuck you" to him by drinking so much. I don't know, I haven't pinpointed it yet, 'cause I've only just got thirty days' sobriety now, and I'm just starting to get some of my memory back.

I mean, I never really had those mornings when you wake up and not know what you were doing the night before. I've woken up and had that feeling for a little while, and then it comes back to me. I've not been lucky enough that I've never had something like that happen to me. I did, one time, go over to my girlfriend's real pissed off, 'cause when I called over there some guy answered the phone. I got all pissed and I was drunk, so I had to go and ride over there and act Mr. Macho. I got there and rang the bell, and this guy opened the door and I slugged him in the face. I found out the next morning it was her brother, and it was like I felt, you know, "Oh, my God." I'm really not, I'm not a violent person. In fact, that's about the only time I ever got into a fight when I was drunk. See, that's why I didn't even remember, because when I was drunk I never really got violent—I kind of got kind of silly and stupid, you know. I mean, that's why I drank—just to get loose.

But I did, I really did, start drinking a lot right about then. I had my own apartment for the first time, and me and the guys would go over there and jam—you know, practice. I had a lot of friends. I still do. Some of them are in a situation like mine now—you know, being addicted and all—and some aren't. I have a lot of friends that are still using, and some that seem like they can take it or leave it. I guess most of them are still using pretty heavy. I wouldn't really suggest that they get into a rehab at all because when it was suggested to me, I said, "Fuck you, you know, you're crazy." You know, though, I never said, "I can stop whenever I want." I never came up with that excuse. I don't know where people got that bullshit excuse. But I would always say, "I don't care, because I like it, you know, it makes me feel good, and I don't mind." I didn't really know whether I was addicted or not, but I didn't think about it either. I didn't. I mean, five years ago nobody could have told me that I'd be like this now, but I probably would've agreed with them just to get 'em off my back. That's the kind of person I was. But in my head I would've said, "Yeah, he's full of shit." 'Cause that could've never happened to me; it's always the next person. But I was drinkin' so much then. I never had anything like where I'd black out for a couple days at a time, but I was drinkin' enough that I know I fried some brain cells along the way. I just read somewhere that, every time you have a drink, something like a couple million cells go, just even on one drink, so I'm probably trillions gone, or something like that.

Being in a band and around other musicians created an environment conducive to drug and alcohol use, which made it easier, for Michael, to get in trouble.

Crank came into the scene in the band too. I thought that was cool, 'cause it was cheaper than coke and it really got you speeded up. So we'd use that. Off and on, mainly before gigs, is when we usually did it. And then sometimes at parties. If it was around, you'd say, "That's fun," but it's not like we went out of our way to get any or anything like that.

One time, when I was real blitzed, I think it was on some crank and booze, I got in a hit-and-run. After I graduated, my dad had bought me this old car, an old Gremlin, and it was a real piece of shit, but it was wheels. Anyway, I had my buddy in the car with me, and we were just coming back from a recording gig that we had done. And it was our first demo tape, and we were all excited and had partied there at the studio. We were coming home, I was dropping him off, and we had to go in this alley, and there was water there. So I was gonna be real bitchin' and spin the tires, right? Well, I spun the whole car around, and it hit this parked car and my buddy jumped out and ran, and I just took off, just drove away. I didn't hit a person, but in the state of mind I was, I would've run if it'd been someone in there too.

**"I just didn't feel comfortable with my surroundings," Michael said when asked what drove him to drink so much. "I did it just to get away."**

I know a lot of people, like the people I've met in rehab, who say they were "turning off their feelings" with alcohol and drugs. Yeah, that's true too for me. When I was real young, I always seemed to keep mostly to myself. I didn't have a lot of friends when I was real young. And the friends that I did have had a couple years on me. I've always made friends of that older crowd. I skipped a grade in school, so right from the beginning I was always the youngest wherever. Even in my band, I was the youngest.

I knew I had a problem with alcohol when I was, like,

eighteen. I really knew I had a problem with alcohol. That's when I finally admitted to myself. But I didn't really mind it then because I was functioning. Which means I had a girlfriend, I had material possessions, and I had the band, so it didn't really create a problem in my life at that time. Except for, you know, acting silly and stupid. Which didn't matter anyways 'cause everybody else was acting silly and stupid 'cause they were wasted half the time too. So I didn't stand out for a long time—at least, I didn't see it that way—until I got hurt.

I was involved in a motorcycle accident which put me in the hospital for about four months when I was just about to turn nineteen. The piece-of-shit car my father gave me had broken down, so I bought this motorcycle and I was on it and some guy hit me—just BAM!—and drove away, and it put me in the hospital. And that helped kind of, 'cause I didn't use when I was in there for about a month and a half. Well, actually, they were shootin' me up with Demerol every four hours, so I was on cloud nine that whole time I was in there; I had a broken leg and severe vascular damage, you know, all the way up. They were gonna amputate me, it was that bad. But then they sent me to this other place, another hospital, where they don't give you a bunch of drugs to ease the pain. They want you to get off the drugs and start learning to deal with the pain. So I didn't use that whole time I was in there. So when I got out of the hospital, I had my cast on, but my mom had lost her condo—she'd declared bankruptcy. She was renting a room from somebody. I had no place to go, is basically what it was. So I applied for GR [General Relief]. And I called my dad, and he started helping me out with rent. But with my leg hurting real bad, well, you know, alcohol's a real good way to ease the pain—plus dealin' with the fact I couldn't do anything. All my friends'd go to places, and go to the beach, and here I am with my broken leg, I can't do nothing. So I basically sat around and got drunk, at least five times out of the week. At least. Sitting alone.

That's when drinking alone started happening. My dad started sending more money, and I was able to drink more. I had also—the week before I had my motorcycle accident—I got arrested for a 502 [Driving under the Influence]. And I had a court date, which I had missed 'cause I was in the hospital, and so I went back to court when I got out of the hospital. My father told me, he said, 'cause he popped bail for me, that he wasn't gonna help me out. He said, "You got yourself into this situation, I'm gonna let you get out." But I think he did help out, 'cause he knew a lot of the judges and people that work in the County, from when I'd got arrested for pot. Anyway, the case is still pending. I have to go back in a few months.

But the drinking went on for the period that I had my cast on. It was about fourteen months from the accident till when I got the cast off. That was a long time. I went back to school in January, and I was doin' okay. I don't know how I was 'cause I was drunk most of the time. Not in school but, you know, after school, I'd go get alcohol. And I don't know how I passed some of my classes. I used my GR money for drinking, and I used my dad's money to pay rent. Then I lost my place because of drinking. At where I was staying, at Steve's place—my friend. It was him and his mother and sister, in a junior one-bedroom. And that's not even a bedroom, that's a wall divider, okay? And they kicked me out because of my drinking. I was hiding bottles, I was hiding bottles through the apartment. Then I decided my aunt would let me come and live with her. It was hard for me to get it into the house and drink 'cause she doesn't work and she's home all the time, so I found ways—come back from school, stop in the liquor store, and drop it off—hide it in the bushes someplace 'cause she was in a condo—and then, when she took her shower and left to go do some errands or something, go downstairs and pick it up and bring it upstairs. I also cleaned out her liquor cabinet. All I did was, I'd sit in my room and listen to tunes. And I also had friends come over that visited me a lot, and we'd drink together too, some of my old drinking buddies, and I was still going out with them and drinking. My aunt really didn't mind, she didn't really think I had a drinking problem at first—until she found her liquor cabinet full of water. 'Cause she didn't drink, that was for guests and stuff. She found out when she had guests come over and she served them water, and it was, like, really embarrassing for her. She got real pissed. I was really close to getting kicked out then. And this is within a month's time.

Then I was kicked out. I finally had come back drunk and she just said to get out of there. So I went to my friend John, the guitar player. That place had a lot of big-time using going on there. And I was living off GR entirely, 'cause my dad stopped sending the checks once I got out of my aunt's, 'cause she told him what I was doing, and he said, "Okay, well, we've had enough of that." So John would let me stay there without paying rent. I just gave him a little bit of money for the electric bill. He had a big house, this big old house, where his father, his sister, and his sister's boyfriend lived. I stayed there for about three months, till I got my brace off my leg. I had no real money to save and buy a car, so I started riding the motorcycle again, which really only got slightly hurt in my accident. I took care of registration and started riding it again. And eventually the motorcycle broke down. And then for sure I had no means of transportation. I was still living off GR, still getting notes from my doctor that I can't work yet. And if I had any pain, he'd send some Tylenol 3's, you know, with codeine. The most I took, I took four at one time once. And I got so buzzed off that I couldn't sleep, and I couldn't do nothing, I just sat and did nothing. That wasn't a good high at all. One or two, it's okay, but four was just a little bit too much, and so I learned quickly from that experience. I also found that drinking beer with codeine was fun too. Me and my friend John would sit around and have the place to ourselves, and we'd pop a couple codeines and drink a six-pack. He had a Prophet 5, which is a synthesizer, that he had bought—me and him had pitched in when we were in the band together—and we'd sit and play music all night off a codeine and beer high.

But this was all going downhill. It was coming to an end fast for me, 'cause I was drinking just about every day then. Coke wasn't in the picture, not much at all, 'cause I didn't have the money. It would've been fine if I, you know, I could afford it or if my friends could afford it. Everyone was really having financial problems. So John's dad decided that they were gonna sell the house and move to this cheaper house, and there's not gonna be enough room for me. So I'm going to these different places, I'm tryin to find a place to rent in exchange for work, right? And that doesn't work, and eventually these people move, and I needed a place to go, and so I called up my mom, and she said, "Well, you can stay here a couple days and, you know, try to find a place. I'll let you use the phone."

Eventually, I found a place to live, and I also found a job that paid two hundred and eighty dollars a week. So I thought, "Oh, this is goin' great, and pretty soon I'll be able to buy another motorcycle." And the first thing that goes in my mind is, I'll be able to afford alcohol and coke again, and everything will be just dandy. I also planned on rippin' off General Relief a little bit longer—as long as I got notes from the doctor, right? So after I got this job, I had come home one night to my mom's, 'cause I had to wait a couple weeks for the other people to move out of this room where I was gonna move into, and I came home wasted, and she said, "Get out of the house!" And from there I went on a drunken spree for a week. Drunk all the time. 'Cause I also just, that same day, I'd got my General Relief check. So I didn't really care, and I just went out and got drunk. I lost the job 'cause I never showed, and I lost the place where I was supposed to live 'cause I never showed. I was so drunk that week I didn't do anything but drink. My basic attitude was, "Fuck it, I'll survive somehow." I didn't care about anything, really, 'cause I was so anesthetized all the time. You don't care, you're feelin' good, you know. The way I was feeling, it would've been okay if I died.

I really did not care whatsoever. I really had no control. I basically started drinking to get—so I wouldn't shake all the time. After a while, I just had to drink every day, otherwise I'd get the DT's. This went on for about a week. Since I had my check and a little bit of money left over from my last check, and I had about a hundred dollars in food stamps, I decided I'm gonna go to one of these cheap, cheap motels—the adult movies and stuff. And this was costing me thirty-five bucks a day. This little piece-of-shit motel was costin' me thirty-five bucks a day. So anyways, I met the neighbors who were renting the room next to me, and they happen to be crack dealers, and he also happens to be a pimp. A couple days later, they decide they have to move. And he had some stuff he had to get rid of and he couldn't pay his rent. So I popped the cash for them—"So long as you pay me back it's cool, you know," that kind of thing—so the pimp caught on to me. He said, "Yeah, this guy's really cool." And he got rid of the stuff, and he paid me back, and he had another dealer bring him some coke in, which was about an ounce—the most coke I've ever seen in my life—and he started having his girl go out and do tricks for him to get money. We got wasted together. We based—the first time I ever based.

But I'm still drinkin' every day. And this went on for about two days. And finally I ran out of money, and, well, he started giving me crack to get rid of. He said, "Well, I'll give you a room, I'll pay your rent here if you can get rid of some of this crack." And that worked for about another two days. And there was always alcohol around, and there was always crack to be smoked, and there was a room for me to stay in. And since I was always stoned and always high, I'm thinkin', "This is the life, you know, what else could I ask, what more could I ask for?" 'Cause I had buddies all over that would come and buy crack, you know. They weren't really buddies, but they were people I had known from different acquaintances; they weren't, like, my friends from junior high or high school. But this went on for about two days.

One day, the pimp guy had left me in the room—he had to go out and make a run, so he left me in the room. He had an ounce in the room with me, hid inside the TV 'cause he took the TV apart—and I had fallen asleep, I passed out. That was, like, the first blackout I can remember ever having, and he thought I took off. He thought I took his stuff and took off. What happened was, he came back and knocked on the door and no one answered. And the lights were out and everything, you know. And he busted the door down, you know. He said later, he told me, he must've been out there for at least twenty minutes knocking. When the door flew open, and he saw me, he goes, "Oh, you fuckin' addict, you passed out and scared the shit out me. I've been out here twenty minutes knockin'." Well, the next thing I know I hear these sirens, and we could see the police comin.' So I split and jumped the wall. Everyone took off. The pimp went one way, and his girl went the other way, and I went out the back and hopped the wall into somebody's backyard, and ran. That's the last I've seen of the pimp.

Next thing I know is, I'm broke. I had food stamps left, that's it. I had no place to stay. I hadn't contacted any of my family in the last two weeks. I was able to steal alcohol from the supermarkets. I found an easy way to do that. So I still had alcohol but I had no place—I was sleepin' on the grass, in front of apartments for about two days, just doing nothing but drinking. I remember the first day, I had my shoes ripped off of me. Someone came with a knife and took my shoes, and took my jacket and my backpack. I had Nikes on, brand-new Nikes that my mom had bought me, you know, when I was staying with her, and he took my shoes and my backpack with all my clothes and stuff in it. So I was bummin' it. I went to the supermarket, ripped off a bottle of plum, apricot, you know—apricot brandy or something—and got drunk, and I was sittin' on the grass. I guess this was the second day, when a guy came up and said, you know, "What's wrong?" I guess he'd seen me with no shoes. I hadn't showered in a couple days, and he took me to his hotel room. And I'm really kind of worried about this guy, but I went anyways. He gave me a meal, he gave me these tennis shoes that I'm wearin' right here. He was a guy who had went through an alcohol program before. And he had just come out of the hospital. He gave me a hundred bucks, and we went out together and bought some new clothes. He was from about fifty miles away, but he had this other business, this insurance business office, near where I was hangin' out, and he had come down to the office to take care of some paperwork. He'd seen me off the street in his car. And I told him, you know, I'd been drinkin', all this and that. He was tellin' me that he'd just got out of a program and: "I've been in your shoes, and I know how you're feelin'."

At first I thought he was some old queer trying to make me or something, but I was drunk enough—you know, fucked up enough—that I didn't care. I did not care about anything at all. I wouldn't have cared if the guy took out a knife and slit my throat, you know. I had no place to go. In fact, I was in such a stupor that I called up General Relief and said, "If you don't find me a place I'm gonna sue you. If you don't find me a place to live, I'm gonna call my attorney and sue you!" But this guy let me drink there; I told him that I needed a drink 'cause I couldn't stand the shaking, and he let me drink. And he wanted to know if I had anyplace to go, and I said no. And he said, "What about your mother and father?" And I said, "Well, they'll have nothing to do with me 'cause of my drinking," and I told him that I thought I would like to find some help but I didn't know how to go about doing it. And that was true—I didn't know how to go about doing it. He said, "Well, we'll try to find you a place. You can use the phone here and I'll give you some numbers, and you can call some of the detoxes and find if you can get a bed, and they'll let you sleep there, and they'll feed you a meal."

And I said okay, 'cause that sounded cool. You know, I was sick and tired. I either got help or I would've been dead.

Well, to make kind of a long story real short, I got put into this great program, and, like I said, it's been thirty days sober for me now. But the desire to go out and drink is still real strong. 'Cause the desires are still with me now. Every day they're with me. They tick in the back of your mind, you know. They tick in the back of your mind.

I'm just gonna take it from there, but you know, these last thirty days have been the best I've probably had. Just being sober. I have more good days now than I did when I was drinking, but there are bad days. But the good days outweigh the bad days by far. You know, when I was drinking, especially when the drinkin' got out of control, there's—you try so many times to get that old fun party-type feeling back, but you never do.

I know so much more than I used to about this stuff. I guess you can't know until you've been through it. My aunt didn't believe I was an alcoholic—she thought I was too young. Then I heard somebody at a meeting say that you're never too young to die.

# KAREN

**"I feel so young to be so old."**

When I was twelve my next-door neighbor had her Bat Mitzvah, so at this big fancy reception she had I was hanging around this guy who was older, and he said, "Let's go get a drink," so I said okay. You know, it was a big catered thing, and I guess the bartender didn't care or what, so this guy ordered us two scotch on the rocks or something. And after that we went around, like taking sips of other people's drinks, people that we knew. You know, "Oh, hey, what are you drinking?" By the end of the night, I was really drunk. And it was great, I was loving every minute of it. It's weird, 'cause I remember that experience so well. It's hard for me to remember when I first started to use but that first time, I remember really well. 'Cause it was like, "God, this is great. I don't feel a thing." I felt great. I went home in the car with the girl whose Bat Mitzvah it was, in her parents' car. I was in the back seat with the other two girls, two sisters, and I kept my mouth shut; I didn't want to talk. I was drunk. If I'd talked I probably would've slurred. So no one knew anything, and when I got home, my parents were asleep, so I just went up to bed. As I started to go to bed, I remember everything spinning, thinking, "Wow." But after a while, it was kinda like, "Okay, stop, you know." I wanted it to stop. And I woke up the next morning and felt okay. I didn't think anything of it. This was definitely the beginning of my getting-loaded career.

The drinking incident, not uncoincidentally, occurred at the time Karen, seventeen at the time of the interview, was

**changing schools—going from middle school to high school. It was a time she remembers as being particularly painful.**

The group that I kind of found myself hanging around was the, quote, bad kids. Which I liked. I was always attracted to, not the kids that did really good—I never really looked up to them, I thought they were all nerds—but the bad kids, the ones that smoked cigarettes behind the buildings, that kind of shit. I was always attracted to that, all my life. I'd always been mommy's or daddy's good little girl. Being the youngest—my brother and sister are a lot older than me—I always kind of was. I was nice. So I was just attracted to that group, to that kind of people, the bad people. You know, I had to get them to like me, though, so I started to get really into punk. I had the creepers, those big shoes, and I had a leather jacket, and I had the Black Flag T-shirts, and then I decided I wanted to do something with my hair. It was short, but I wouldn't settle for anything longer than shaved at that time. So I went and shaved it, got a Mohawk. I did it at home, and when my mom came home, she flipped out: "What did you do to your hair, you're letting it grow, I'm taking away all your razors and all the scissors out of the house"; she just freaked. And I just kind of said, "But I like it, it's cool, Mom." She works for an orthodontist, so she's like, "Well, I see kids all day, and none of 'em have come in there with that." So that's what happened. I remember thinking that I always wanted to be rebellious, yet at the same time I didn't want my parents to get angry at me for making my hair like that, cutting my hair like that. It was kinda like, "Just leave me alone. Just let me do my thing."

For a long time me and my mom did not get along at all, and I would just stay in my room all the time. I lived with my mom. My parents are divorced. In fact, they'd just gotten a divorce right before this. Yeah, that's right, I was still twelve. And when my dad saw it, saw my hair—

my dad is real different from my mom, my dad's, like, laid back, kicked back—he's like, "Well, do you like it?" And I said yeah. He said, "Well, that's nice, you know, as long as you like it." I saw him about twice a week then, like one night after school and then on Sundays. Typical divorce arrangement.

Karen's friendships with the "bad" kids quickly introduced her to pot smoking.

I don't remember feeling anything my first time I smoked, but everyone told me that's normal. I used to see everyone stoned, and they'd laugh and they were having fun and I thought, "God, give me some of that." And plus, they were the bad kids again. And they always seemed to be happy, they always had friends, always had friends. And the school like kinda looked up to them, like no one would mess with them. It's a real small group, but like everyone knows them at the school. It was like, if I hadn't met those people, though, I probably would've not done it. Maybe, I don't know, I can't really tell. I do remember one thing, it stands out: I told a couple people, "Yeah, I got so drunk at my next-door neighbor's," and they were, like, laughing, "Oh, that's cool, you know," so it made me feel accepted, 'cause they thought that was cool and they were laughing. "Your friend's Bat Mitzvah and you got drunk," and they thought that was real funny.

We'd go out on weekends and we'd smoke pot and drink. It was either our parents' alcohol—"Let's take a bottle out of my parents'" or someone would—or we'd hang out at liquor stores and wait for people to walk by and we'd go, "Are you over twenty-one, can you buy us a six-pack of whatever?" We did that all the time. We had our ways.

For a long time, I think until I was about fourteen, pot and alcohol were the only drugs I did. I still had weird-color clothes, weird haircuts, you know. I used to have a black mohawk with white at the tips, and I let it grow a little bit, just so you could barely pull it, and I did that white, like blond, same color as the top, you know; I was messing with colors and stuff like that. I did bad in school, which is another weird thing, 'cause I'm really smart, I really am, and I'd always gotten good grades before. I didn't like authority figures, I was real anti-authority, you know, like, "You're not gonna tell me what to do." There was a long period of time when me and my friend Jenny—she lived about three miles from my house—would meet at about seven-fifteen in the morning, before school, and we'd go back in this little place by the school, these bushes, everyone called it "the hole." There was like all these bushes and there's the circle of old rocks, then there's houses, and we used to party back there before school; we used to smoke pot—we called 'em seven-fifteens, and we'd talk on the phone so our parents wouldn't catch on: "Yeah, we'll do seven-fifteens tomorrow." My mom would wonder why I left so early for school, and I'd tell her it was to go study. I don't know why she believed me. I'd say, "Oh, I'm gonna get there a little early and go to the library." So we'd go there and get stoned in the morning, come to school high, you know, and then in between second and third periods there's nutrition, and we'd go in the bathroom then and get high. We'd be in the stall and we'd bend down. Everyone who smoked in the bathrooms had a password. When the aides came in, we'd say, "What time is it?" so everyone would throw their joints in the toilet. Between all the cigarette smoke, though—you were allowed to smoke in the bathrooms—you couldn't smell the weed, really, especially 'cause the ladies that came in the bathrooms to check, you could probably show 'em a bag of weed and they wouldn't know what it was. So we'd take a few hits, you know. Or, the best, what we used to do is, we'd time it in class, when we were both gonna take the hall pass and go to the bathroom and meet there, 'cause usually no one ever comes in the bathroom during class. And then at lunch, we'd leave. They were building these houses around the block from the school, so we'd go in these unbuilt houses. We had our own room and everything, and we'd sit up there with a whole bunch of people and smoke pot.

Once a good student, Karen was now getting only D's and F's.

I ended up going to summer school to do some of the ninth grade over again. I just didn't care about school. I'd stopped caring. I only went 'cause of my parents, 'cause they were on my case. All I wanted to do was just be left alone. I didn't want my parents on my case, I just wanted to be left alone to get high. So if I went to summer school, they couldn't say anything. All I wanted to do was graduate and be on my own. I had real attitude problems towards them. I think they were, like, thinking that I was going through a phase, which I kept telling them, "Yeah, I'm just going through a phase." My mom would tell me to do something, and I'd roll my eyes. Anything she said to me I was like gonna take the other side, or get defensive about it, or fight. It was like, I just didn't even want my mom to talk to me.

My father spoiled me. He still does. I was always real nice to Dad. He always gave me money. That was how he showed me he loved me. My mom never gave me money, really. She always told me to get money from Dad. You know, they were at each other's throats for a long time after they got divorced. And it was like, "Tell your father to buy you that, tell your father to give you money." I guess they used me as a weapon between them. I was like the little message carrier sometimes too, like, Mom says that she needs whatever. 'Cause they were still, like, dividing all this property they had and, like, stocks and bonds, so I was kinda like, "Mom wants this," and my dad would say, "Well, tell your mother that." They talked through me, 'cause when they talked directly to each other, they fought. And if I happened to be there, then they'd say, "Well, that's easier than talking on the phone," so they'd go through me a lot too, as well as argue on the phone all the time. My sister was about fifteen years old, and my brother twelve years older, so they were both long gone out of the house by the time all this happened. I guess basically I was kind of an only child. My mom worked full-time, two jobs, so she wasn't home a lot. You know, I never told them to stop using me like that. I don't know why. I think part of it may be because it hurt too much, and I couldn't, you know, I didn't know how to express. I didn't know I was hurt at the time, and I didn't know how to express it, so I just shoved it in; I just kept swallowing the hurt that I had. They never asked me how I felt. The only time something like that was asked was when they asked me who I wanted to live with. I said, "Mom, in the house." I like my dad better—at least, I got along with him better—but I wanted to stay because of the neighborhood. My dad lived in various condos for a while till he settled down again.

**Not surprisingly, considering they had no idea how the bitterness in their divorce was affecting their daughter, Karen's parents didn't suspect she was drinking and smoking pot.**

I bought pot a lot. But usually we always had it, someone always had it. Whether it was me or Jenny or any of the other people, we always had weed, and we got to be real good friends with the people that sold it to us. That way, we'd get good prices and we'd get it before it had gone through fifteen other people taking little bits out; we'd get it right from the resource.

When I was fourteen, about mid-fourteen, I decided that alcohol and weed were great together—separately, in combination, all at once, everything. And a lot of my friends started to do coke. My best friend, Jenny, she had been doing it for a while, but I just never did it. Not because—if it was there, I would have done it. But she did it with her boyfriend, mainly 'cause he always had it. And then one day, I was over at Jenny's. See, her house is where I always was because her parents smoked pot, and so does her brother. Her parents were, like, freaks—they grew up in the sixties, like nature freaks. And they always had it, so Jenny sometimes stole it from them. And they probably knew that Jenny was smoking it, but they didn't care, 'cause *they* did, so they didn't see anything wrong with it, I guess. So we were always at Jenny's, so we could party in her room, or just go outside. We always just stayed there till real late, 'cause her parents used to go out till real late, and we'd just party. One time I was over there when her parents were out real late, and her boyfriend, Carl, had some coke. I said, "Okay, I'll do it." I wasn't scared or anything, and I snorted it. I didn't like coke so much, I never did, all through my using. I never liked coke, I just didn't like the feeling, I didn't like being so—that feeling in your stomach, and you smoke two packs of cigarettes in two hours, you know. You wake up feeling terrible the next morning. I just thought: Mornings, it was so natural to wake up and feel like shit. I'd just wake up, I'd feel like shit, so I'd grab a joint, smoke it, and I'd feel better. But this first time, doing coke, it made me less scared of a lot of other things—acid and all that—which a lot of the people were doing too.

Getting to know Carl and his friends was a big step. They were even better than our friends: they had more drugs, big and better things, so that was even better. I took pills, I took downers and uppers, Christmas Trees, Cross-Tops. If I couldn't find any pills, I'd take, like, thirteen Dexatrim, which—God, I learned my lesson real quick with those. Or I'd take No-Doz, a bunch of No-Doz to, you know, get up. Plus, starting to hang around Jenny's house all the time, getting to know her older brother and his friends, we started hanging around older people. And we'd walk around school like—we'd sell to the stupid rich girls that didn't know anything; we'd make a lot of money off them, 'cause they didn't know what they were doing. We'd sell 'em a dime bag that was about five dollars worth, and we'd sell 'em parsley or something stupid like that, to make money for our drugs. And then, what really started me getting going was my brother moved back home. Now, my brother and my sister are real different; they're like two totally different role models. My sister always did real good in school, then got married—she's just like a good kid, she always has been. Sure, she experimented and stuff with drugs. But that was just a small part of her life, and my mom always wanted me to grow up just like her. My brother's, like, the black sheep of the family. He did real good in high school, got straight A's. But when he was seventeen, he stole, just out of the blue—I don't know why he did this, 'cause he's such a smart kid, he graduated high school at sixteen—five thousand dollars from my parents and went to England for a week. Then he came back and said, "Thanks for the vacation." It was amazing. My parents had had this cash in the envelope that they were saving for a vacation for them, and he just took it and flew off for a week. He said he had a great time. My brother does everything, all kinds of drugs. He never went to college. I mean, he went for about a month and dropped out. I don't know what it was. When he came back to live with us, it was 'cause he had run out of money. He'd been everywhere: hitchhiked across the country and lived in Wyoming for a while, lived in the Sierras for a while; like being a cook, just little jobs. And he came back, and he was a born-again Christian all of a sudden, a Jesus freak. I think he had a lot of resentments against my parents, 'cause they shoved Judaism down his throat, both my sister and my brother. With me, they gave up on it.

And my brother came into town, and I guess he could tell that I smoked weed—just the way I'd come in—and I knew my brother did, but we never approached each other for a few months. And then we did, and we started to party together. And so I'd get drugs from my brother and his friends. And I'd buy, like, sixty dollars worth, three eighths, and then sell it and make more money and buy more—while I was supporting my habit. My brother's dealer was this big bouncer guy, and he wouldn't let me meet him for a long time; he wouldn't tell me his name, where he lived, nothing. But finally when I met him, I started to sell weed for him, because I was young, and I was making a lot of money off the rich stupid kids. You know, they always had a bunch of money on them, and I'd make profit. So then I started to think I was tough shit, that I was bad. And I started ditching school. I'd go to school to socialize or to sell. I wasn't going to school for school. I mean, I wasn't really before that, but it was worse, much worse. And everyone knew me as a stoner—a punk. But I also hung around long-hair people, like rock 'n' roll heavy-metal-type people.

My mom had been dating this guy for two years, and he was great. I loved him. I was real close with him. He was real cool when I dyed my hair hot pink or whatever color—orange or whatever color it was. He said, "Hey, that's cool." He was a real cool guy. I loved him. He accepted me, or that's what I thought. He probably did. But he had a sudden heart attack and died. He was forty-two fuckin' years old. He died right in front of me and my mom, right there. He had had a bad heart before that, and he was diabetic. And he had these little insulin patches that he used to wear, and he had his little insulin shoot-up kit. And he had a bad heart. And after that, that's when I really flipped out. My mom was going through a hard time. I couldn't stand—I'd wake up in the middle of the night and hear my mom cry, and I hated being at home, 'cause my mom was going through hard times, I was going through hard times. Here she was, having this man die on her, still having two jobs, trying to support everyone. And that's when I flipped out. And I was real into self-destruction. And I was real suicidal.

I started going to a therapist; my mom took me to a

therapist, and my dad paid for it. And I was real honest with her, with the therapist, except when it came to drugs. I didn't tell her I did drugs. I never went there high. I'd smoke pot up until an hour before I had to go, 'cause I didn't want to be loaded when I went there. I really respected her. She was, like, the only person I respected when I was getting loaded, I guess because it was someone who I could let see who I was. Which I didn't. I didn't let anyone see who I really was inside. I didn't know even who I was. At school and anywhere else I'd dress in all black. Which would push people away, and I'd push people away. I always felt that I didn't fit in with anyone. In fact, I think I had that feeling ever since I was about twelve. I always felt I was a lot more mature than a lot of people my age, maybe because my brother and sister were so much older.

I always used to hang around people that were older than me. But even then, I never really felt like I fit in, probably because I didn't let myself fit in; I didn't let them get to know me so they could accept me and let me in, basically. But I didn't know that was the problem. 'Cause I could be around a certain group of people and act that way, and I could be around a different group and act this way, and none of them are me. That's how I always felt. And I used to tell that to my therapist. I was real open with her, except about drugs; I didn't tell her about my drug habit, which was a pretty big part of me, yeah, but I was afraid she was gonna tell someone, even though I knew she couldn't say anything to my parents, about anything that we talked about, unless I told her she could. But eventually I did, but I told her that I smoked pot once in a while—I didn't tell her it was every day, all day, every day. I had to tell her something, 'cause it was bothering me. It was almost like I couldn't keep it from her. So while all this was going on, I remember, one night, I was sitting in my room and I was really depressed. And I went into the bathroom and I got two razor blades and I put 'em in my room, and I said, "Okay, I'm gonna kill myself right now." And so I put on a punk album. I used to say I liked the words; it was like, "Fuck authority, fuck everything." And I slit my wrists up and down the vein, and I was crying, I was hysterical, and I ran out crying, hysterical. My mom was in the other end of the house, and I showed her what I'd done: I just held out my wrists. Well, she freaked out and called my therapist, who told her to take me to the hospital right now. I wanted to go, 'cause I didn't want to go cut myself more. For some reason, I wanted to go in the hospital; when she said that, I was, like, glad. I wanted to go. I was so deranged. I had so many drugs in my system. I was always either on drugs or coming off them. There wasn't a single day for at least the last year when I didn't get high on something. If I didn't smoke pot at lunch at school, I was entirely a bitch. I didn't want to talk to anyone. All I wanted to do was smoke weed. Alcohol I could do without, but I had to have pot. I used to smoke it with opium too, sometimes. Sometimes we didn't even know, and then we'd smoke it, and, "Oh, there's opium in this." I was just completely deranged.

I remember, it was like three in the morning when we got there and checked me in and stuff. By then, it had sort of stopped bleeding. They cleaned it up, put on bandages, and it wasn't, like, spurting out or anything. They made me strip down to naked, to make sure I didn't have anything on me. They took away my lighter; my mom had found out by this time that I smoked cigarettes. That was like her big . . . She found 'em or something, and she said, "I don't want you to smoke," and she took them away. "And if I ever see cigarettes . . ." You know, I tried to tell her, "Mom, please, I smoke," 'cause to me that was like a nothing. But to her it was a big thing, 'cause she didn't know about anything else. So they stripped me down. I didn't have any drugs with me, but they took away my lighter, not the cigarettes.

I was in a room with this other girl. And I was sitting there, and the nurse was cleaning me up, and I was sitting on the bed just looking around, and the girl next to me woke up. She looks at me and she goes, "Who the fuck are you?" And I just go, "I'm Karen." And she had like a cast on her leg, and she was just a real bitch. She was just like, "Who the fuck are you? Get out of here," she said to me, "get out of here. I'm trying to sleep. Turn off the fuckin' light," and all this stuff, and I'm just listening to her. I didn't say anything to her. I was just like, "Yeah, whatever." And then they cleaned me up, gave me their little pajamas, and after I did all this paperwork, I talked to a couple of the people working there—therapists, I guess—and I just remember going to sleep, like, laying there in bed.

For some reason, I didn't eat for, like, two, two-and-a-half days. And they kept trying to make me eat, but I just didn't want to eat. I didn't want to be there; I did, but I didn't. I was real into self-destruction, so I'd throw up once in a while, but not like all the time. I wasn't ever bulimic. Not eating, I guess, was the only weapon I had against their authority. I guess a lot of people, a lot of the girls and guys, that go in there do the same thing. That's what they told me. So they kinda let me run my little trip. And then I went in and ate. And they knew I'd eat. When it stopped getting me attention, I started to eat. I was in there for four weeks, and they never knew I had a drug problem. They never figured out that my slitting my wrists might have had something to do with drugs; they never took blood tests or anything, and they thought it was just all mental. I was just so screwed up inside, I thought about drugs all the time, but I didn't have any, until this guy Henry came in. He was, like, he seemed really cool, and we were talking one day, and he goes, "Come here for a second," in his room, and he opened up this shoebox filled with joints, and it was just like he was my friend. He was my best friend that day. And in fact, I remember one time we were in his room, and we stood up on the toilet, 'cause there was a vent on the top by the toilet, so we stood up on the toilet seat and we were smoking this joint, blowing the smoke through the vent. Well, we found out later in the day that the smoke had traveled through and gone out the last room in the corridor, and it was a cop's room, and there was a cop standing there, I guess. So they questioned him for weed and all this stuff, 'cause I guess they smelled it or something, but we never got caught. We laughed at that.

I wanted to get real, I really did, but I never did in the hospital. I'd call my friends, and I'd go, "I'm in a hospital." They're like, "What?" And I'd go, "Well, I freaked out last night, you know." And none of them came to visit me, which shows how good friends they really were. What I wanted was just to let down my defenses. I wanted to stop, 'cause it wasn't me. But I wanted to be . . . It wasn't a conscious decision to be a bad kid, and it wasn't a conscious decision to be myself. It was just, I guess I was so sick of my image, and so sick of putting on a show for everyone. That's what I thought I was doing: just people-pleasing. I was a real people-pleaser. You know, I was always really nice; that's all anyone ever said about me: "Karen is so nice." 'Cause I'd pleased everyone except me. You know, I'd give my right arm, basically, except when it came to drugs—then I was selfish, and all of that. If I wanted to party with someone I'd turn 'em on for free, 'cause I always had it. But still, I was pretty selfish with it. It took me, at this point, a lot to get stoned; I'd have to smoke a lot of weed to get stoned, not just three or four hits.

Karen eventually became friendly with her roommate, Laura, who, at eighteen, was four years her senior.

Laura knew what she was talking about when it came to punk and music, and she went to a lot of gigs [rock clubs with live music], and I liked that. She used to say, "Yeah, I did acid," and she used to do PCP and shoot heroin and all that. She was there, I guess, 'cause she tried to kill herself too, I don't know. And I really liked that. I'd go, "Wow, you smoked PCP, wow, you shot heroin, that's so cool." I thought that was really cool, and so I got really close to her; not close like we'd talk, but we hung around a lot, and we kept in touch when she left the hospital. She used to call me at the hospital, and she came to see me once, and I asked her, I said, "Are you staying sober?" She goes, "Hell, no, I partied the first day I got out." And I was like, "Cool!" Then I couldn't wait to get out.

And so in the hospital I didn't really grow much or do much of anything. I hardly remember the whole time. It was kinda like a retreat for me—you know, I slept. And I got out of the hospital, and I was nicer to my mom; we got along a little bit better. She was a lot more like lenient. She was like, okay, she didn't want me to do that again, you know. She probably thought it was all her fault. And you know what? I can't believe I did that, but I tried to tell her it was, that it was her fault. So she had a lot of guilt. And she said, "I don't want you hanging around the old people." So I said okay. But I did anyway, and I still kept talking to Laura, and she lived about forty miles away, so I ran away once. And I met her. I used to take the bus to Hollywood a lot, just to go see the punks and walk on the avenue and stuff like that. And so I met her one day, and I ran away for the weekend and stayed up there. We went to gigs, you know, saw punk bands play. I was only fifteen, so my mom sent the police out looking for me, but I came home in a couple days. She figured that I ran away, 'cause I used to threaten to do it all the time. God, I can't believe the things I did to my mom. Lot of guilt, still, now, even now.

That weekend I ran away I tried acid for my first time. I was scared for a while. I was scared while I was on it, you know, 'cause Laura and her friends all knew what they were doing. But they thought it was cool, 'cause I was so much younger than them. "Oh, let's get little Karen blazed, let's see her get wasted." I mean, they all took it too. But they had been used to it, sort of, you know, tried it lots of times before.

That was scary. I couldn't control myself like I could when I was stoned. But the thing is, that's exactly what I was looking for. I mean, it totally took me away from reality, whereas pot was just a little bit. Watching all these people, these punks at the clubs, you know, I was totally—I didn't know what I was doing, I didn't know where I was, things were moving, the walls would breathe, I'd see trails, you'd move your cigarette and I thought it was a whole bunch of bumblebees or fireflies going like that. That's what I thought it was. But I liked it. From the very first time I tried it I loved it, because it totally took me away from everything. I mean, I felt nothing. No body, right?

I came home and all I wanted to do was take a shower and get something to eat. And I looked at my mom like she was crazy when she started yelling at me, asking me where the hell I was. I said, "That's none of your fucking business. Just leave me alone, I'm tired." I wanted to eat, sleep, and shower, that's what I wanted to do when I got home. I didn't want my mom to talk to me or anything. I used to wonder, "Why can't she just leave me alone? Why?" And my mom used to tell me, "It's just 'cause I care." I'd go, "Bullshit, if you cared you'd leave me alone." And so she came up to give me a hug, just because I was okay, I came home alive, I was alive, you know? And I just sat there like nothing. I went, "Yeah." And I went to my room. Cold. Ice cube. And I called Jenny and I said, "I blazed this week." She goes, "Oh, did you like?" And I said yeah, and she goes, "That's cool. You know what you should try then? You'll fuckin' love it. You have to 'shroom. You have to take mushrooms. That is so much fun." So I'm all, "Okay, you know."

And I was still going to school and everything, even though I was still gettin' F's. And some D's. And me and Jenny still—seven-fifteens and that whole smoking-pot thing was still going on. It's like I'd progressed, but I didn't stop what I was doing before either. I guess I just broadened my drug horizons. So the next weekend after the acid I was sleeping over at Jenny's that night, so I didn't have to worry about a curfew, and we did the 'shrooms. And I liked them even better than the acid—except, I remember, it made me feel really like powerful or really strong. I could crush anything, I could do anything, I could fly if I wanted to. I mean, not literally, but kind of. And I remember looking at this rock, and this rock for some reason looked so pretty to me; it was like purplish-green, it was weird. So I picked it up and I put it in my pocket, and I remember waking up the next morning and my hip hurt, 'cause I'd slept in my pants, and I was like, "God, what's in my pocket?" And it's this stupid ugly rock. And I remembered the night before. I'm going, "Oh, God," and I threw it outside. So I had this bruise right on my hipbone. You know, "What the hell's in my pocket? This stupid rock. Oh, yeah." 'Cause everyone thought it looked neat. They're like, "Keep it," like it was Kryptonite or something.

Starting from that night, I 'shroomed a lot. And one night I did acid. I laughed, laughed all the time. Acid—I think, probably 'cause it was such a bad experience, you know, being at a gig—was, like, very scary to me. But 'shrooms wasn't that scary. Also, 'cause I was around Jenny or people I knew better, it was a lot better. And so we, me and Jenny, we smoked pot, we 'shroomed together, everything. And I did acid here and there over about a five-month period. If booze was around I'd drink it. I remember one time, me and Jenny didn't have anything, nothing but alcohol; we had this, it was called Old Mother's Kentucky Whiskey, or something like that—a hundred proof. We were at my house, and we didn't have a ride to her house through the canyons, so we decided we'd walk. So we started walking along this real deserted highway and stopped at our high school. It was real late, so school wasn't in or anything. It was a weekend, and we started to drink there, 'cause we were cold, so we'd drink to get warm. And we walked all the way to her house, you know, and we sat there and we finished the whole bottle, without standing. We were just sitting there the whole time talking—and by this time it was like drinking water. We were chugalugging it, no problem. By the time we stood up, I think we were so oblivious, we were past the passing-out point. I don't know how we didn't pass out. But, I mean, we stood up, we could not stand, and we threw up our guts. That's the only time I ever threw up alcohol. I mean, it was just insane. Both of us. I thought I was gonna die. I kept going, "Jenny, I'm gonna die." Her brother came home, and he was like, "God, you guys are wasted." He looks at the bottle and it was empty. "Did you drink all this?" And we're like, "Uh-huh." And then we crashed, we went to bed.

When you used to get in trouble at school, they had these things called Saturday work-something, where you go on a Saturday from like nine to twelve to help the janitors clean up. They were called a Saturday work program, that's what it's called. Like the movie *The Breakfast Club*, that kind of thing. And Jenny had one, so we had to be at school at eight. We'd show up because all the bad kids always had those. We'd get in trouble so we'd smoke and party. The janitors would say, "You guys, na-na-na," and we'd hide, we'd party, you know. And the janitors weren't exactly—they probably knew. They saw me and Jenny with it once, they'd let us smoke cigarettes, you know. So we got up the next morning and we were—I don't know how we woke up, I don't know how we made it. So Jenny's mom took us to the high school, and I had to walk home, up this hill from the high school to my house. And my stomach was just, I was just like, I could hardly, I was gone, I was dead, I was like a zombie. So I'm walking home up this hill, and I remember, I started to feel like I was gonna throw up again, so it was on these people's lawn, and I remember this man, I looked up, and this man was, like, looking out their bedroom window on a nice sunny morning, and he sees this kid barfing on his lawn. There I was, I was throwing up, and he's, like, looking at me. I just, I didn't even care. I was afraid he was gonna come out and say something to me, something like, "Clean it up," but he didn't.

Such scenes of excess became a regular part of Karen's life for the next several months. She was now sixteen.

I came home from school one day and I threw my backpack on the table and went in my room, and my mom came into my room holding a bag of weed. She'd found it in my backpack. And she held it up. She said, "Is this yours?" And I said, "Yeah," and I instantly started to cry. I like broke down in front of my mom and I told her I had a drug problem, right then and there. I literally broke down. I told her I wanted help, I told her I needed help. And she said, "Okay, we'll find you help," and I said, "Yes, please find me help." And I watched her dump out all my weed, and I helped her dump it out, except I had another whole thirty dollars worth in my bra at the time. I didn't tell her about that. I thought, "Well, I might need this." So I didn't tell her about that. I watched her dump out what she had found and I told her I needed help, but I wasn't that ready to stop, okay?

Because of her failing grades and because she'd been caught stealing, Karen had been forced to transfer to another school.

One of my friends—well, she wasn't really a friend, but I knew her, and I used to have to take P.E. with her. And I remember this girl had just got for her sixteenth birthday or something this real nice diamond ring with jewels all over it, and she put it up on top of the lockers. She was getting dressed and everything and no one was looking, and I looked at that ring, and I said, "Ah, that ring has gotta be worth bucks." So I took it, took the ring. And I knew this girl. It didn't bother me that I was fucking her over, that she'd just got this. Anyway, I got caught and had to give the ring back, and I guess that did something to my brother, 'cause he went and told my mom which one of my friends—that all my friends partied. He told my mom that Jenny was a bad influence. And at the time I hated him for doing that. He said, he came up to me and he said, "You have to stay sober now, I'm not gonna sell to you anymore."

Then my mom told me they called this drug rehab place, and I went in for a screening. I had real short—real, real short, and you could just barely pinch it—dyed blue-black hair. I was still wearing all black, always a black leather jacket. I looked like a guy; you couldn't really tell if I was a guy or a girl—my bangs covered half my face and were down over my eyes, and I always wore just this disgusting blue-black color. And I walked in and I remember seeing these kids, and I was thinking, "Oh, God," you know, I hated every one of 'em. I didn't even know them. And they were laughing. I was sitting there, and my mom was in talking with the counselors and I was sitting there. I'd smoked a cigarette and I remember I was so insecure. I didn't know it at the time, but I was so insecure. These people intimidated the shit out of me, and I didn't realize it at the time, so I just hated 'em. They knew each other. They didn't know me, I didn't know them. I was always a real insecure person. I hated myself. To me, they were like goody-two-shoes people. So I went in and I talked to the counselor, and for some reason, it didn't occur to me that I was gonna have to stop totally, and I said to her, I said, "Wait, the kids here, they don't do anything?" She said nope, nothing. And I said, "Never?" I thought I'd be able to come here and smoke pot, like, maybe once a week. They told me to come and start groups in a week. That was only a screening.

I told all my friends I was going to a drug rehab and they were like, "Yeah, right!" 'Cause I was like the last one that would get sober, you know? I went home and I still had that weed, and that lasted me for a week, and then I came to this group, the very first group. And I was listening, and I was really listening. It was about eighteen kids in here. We had group, and at the end—and I was listening—all these kids, they looked like kids I'd see at school and stuff, they were talking feelings. I didn't even know *how* to feel. You know, they were talking feelings and they were talking so honest and they were swearing, and I like kept looking at the counselors when they'd swear. And I liked this place when I first went. And I even remember I shared at the end of my first group and said, "God, I can't believe what I'm hearing, you know, this is how I used to get with my therapist." Well, maybe not to that extent, but it was real. And these kids were being themselves. I was impressed. And intimidated. And scared. Real scared. 'Cause I didn't know—didn't want to know—who I was, and I didn't want to know what kind of feelings I had inside of me.

So I came home that night after group. We had this hall in my house, where there's a kitchen on one end and then there's the bedrooms. So my brother was sitting in the kitchen, and you couldn't see the rest of the kitchen, just that part, where he was sitting. And I was standing in the hall, 'cause my mom was over here in the kitchen, so my mom couldn't see when I went to my brother and said, "Do you have any weed?" Well, he turns around and he goes, "Mom, Karen just asked me for weed." And I went, "Oh, God." My mom comes in the hall, and I went, "Oh, sorry, you know. Just a habit." 'Cause I didn't have any. And I stayed sober that day. That was my first day, and I stayed sober, from that point on, for nine months. It wasn't easy, but I did it.

Since I switched schools I didn't hang out much with Jenny anymore, but I still talked to her and stuff, but only a little. Actually, I got to be real close with one of the guys in the program. We were into the same kind of music, and we dressed weird. I'm not sure who I was staying sober for when I first came in the program, because it wasn't for me. Maybe it was for him, 'cause I wanted to be friends with him. Me and my mom gradually started to get along better. Things started to happen for me good, for the first time in years. Since I was twelve. My head was clear for the first time in years. But what I did was, I stayed sober, but I ran from my feelings in every other possible way besides getting loaded. I remember when I first got my car. They wouldn't let me get my car till I had six months sober. So on my six months sober I got my car—that's another thing that was keeping me to stay sober. First day I got my car, I stayed out all night and didn't call my mom. You know, I kept running, and I kept doing bad things.

So I was still running from feelings and running from me, but I wasn't using drugs to do it. And that lasted nine months. And after nine months I got loaded. I was over at a friend's house after school, and I got to know people at my new high school really well. It was with a new group of kids. They weren't addicts. They used drugs, but they didn't talk about it a lot. They did okay in school. It was a better crowd. And so I was over at a friend's house after school one day, and she knew I was sober but to her it didn't mean anything. She didn't understand that I had a real bad problem before, that I was an addict. She was not an addict, just a casual user. And she said, "Do you want to get high?" I don't know what made me do it, but I smoked weed that day. Actually, I do know why: I'm an addict, and if it's there I'll do it. People used to tell me that sobriety has a way of ruining your partying, you know? And I used to say, "If I'm ever gonna slip"—that's what they call it, you slip—"if I'm ever gonna slip, I'm gonna do something real big; I'm gonna take acid, or I'm gonna just get wasted." So I got high. I wasn't like really stoned, I was high. And I just felt so guilty. I came back to the program the next day and I cried, and I told everyone what I'd done. I said: "I used, I slipped, you know, I had nine months sober." And I was real scared. See, I remember, after I came down, I saw myself, I pictured myself like sitting on this wall, one leg over each side, and on this side is all my old friends, just getting loaded and all that, that whole life, and this other side are the right people to hang around. And I chose the right way. You know, it wasn't like a conscious decision, like I sat there and said I'm gonna do this. I just kinda thought about it.

That was the last run I took. After that I really put down my walls and dropped my image and got honest, and that guy that I was real good friends with, he was sober for a year and a half, and he went out and got loaded. And that was real scary too, because he was my support for a long time; I didn't get close with anybody but him. So when he left I felt kind of like I didn't belong almost. That same old feeling. But I started to get close with other people. For the first time, I wanted to do good things for me, I wanted to feel better. Before, I didn't think I deserved it, and any time I'd have a little bit of success I'd screw it up for myself by staying out all night or by getting loaded. I hated myself, I didn't think I deserved to be happy. I didn't know who I was. I felt like I was being shit on by everyone all my life. Like my stepdad, that man my mom was seeing for two years. They never got married but he lived with us, so when he died, I basically felt betrayed.

Then what happened was, my friend Laura, when I first got sober, she thought it was real cool, that I was getting sober. But a couple weeks later, she killed herself. She committed suicide. She took a gun to her head. Then I found out that a couple other people had died in a car accident, a couple of those punkers I knew through her. And I felt, I felt like the time when my kitten ran away. I just always felt like people were leaving me—constantly.

I feel so young to be so old.

# VIC

**"There's most of those two years I don't even remember. They're just a blank."**

In grade school, the cops would come by with their briefcase, showin' all the different kind of drugs. They looked so terrible and scary. You'd say to yourself, "Wow, don't use these. Oh, I'll never. I'd never start smoking cigarettes, that's terrible. Marijuana, that's, that's sick." And then, you know, it just happened. Somebody hands you a joint and there it goes. "Here, smoke this." And it's peer pressure, kind of, wanting to be in with the cool crowd or whatever, to be in their little clique. So I'll just try it this once, you know, and then wham—that was it. That's all it took, the first one. I was gone. People told me, you know, that marijuana will get you into heroin, and cocaine, and lead to all these harder drugs. And I said it never could do that. But it did—led me right in, right into it. Within, within, six months. Within six months, I was just full-blown: alcohol, cocaine, heroin, you name it.

It didn't matter what it was. If I felt bad, I wanted to feel good; if I felt good, I wanted to feel better. So I took drugs. The thing was, it never felt as good as it did the first time I got high. But I just kept doing it anyway. After a while, I didn't get high anymore, they just made me feel like shit. But since I didn't want to deal with anything, I wanted to just keep stuffing those feelings back down inside, I had to take more and more drugs. I used drugs to get out of feeling anything.

Vic, seventeen, smoked marijuana for the first time on his fifteenth birthday. He had never been high on anything before that day, but it would be a long time again until a day he wasn't.

I'd go to a party and have two beers. Two or three would get me drunk. And then the next weekend I'd go for six. And then the next party it would be a case. Just like with pot, you start getting used to alcohol, your body starts building a tolerance, so you take different ones, more of something else, or you start mixing them—trying always to achieve that first high, the first high I ever had. And it never worked. I was smoking, probably on average, a gram of good strong Sinsemillian pot every day for two years trying to get that first feeling back. When your body's goin' through changes, like in puberty, all of that stuff infringes. Oh, it screws up your whole body. Believe me, I was real messed up. I'm still tryin' to get even.

I was drinking a lot and smoking a lot of pot, but at least the drinking was just on the weekends. And then I started taking liquor from my parents' liquor cabinet and drinking before school. I'd get up and, you know, have the shakes or whatever, so I'd drink some alcohol to just make me feel just right. And sometimes during school, I'd bring a thermos full of Kool-Aid or whatever and mix it with whatever I could. At lunch, if I started feeling shaky, I'd drink.

I got terrible grades in school. I've always been an underachiever. They told me I had the potential to be a straight-A student. But I never was, not even before drugs. I got C's, B's at best. But then when I started using, my grades went straight to shit.

Vic's parents had a sour marriage for as long as he could remember, yet he said he was reluctant to blame his home life for his desire to be high constantly. His father was himself an alcoholic, and ironically, while his relationship with his father has improved dramatically since both entered recovery programs, his mother, he said, feels left out and estranged from him.

I started using coke. A friend just said, "Here, try some of this." So I tried it. I snorted it. And I loved it. I mean, it was the best, you know, the best, right there. It made me feel good. But it was real expensive, so I had to, you know, start stealing or dealing or whatever. Before, I had a job cleaning an office. And that would bring in a little money. But other times I would steal from my mom's or my sister's purse. Sometimes out of their rooms. I'd steal from friends, too—either their money or their drugs. I'd get drugs any way I could. Any way I could. I got in just real bad. I stole cars, TVs, radios, jewelry, guns, anything. Break into houses and sell the shit to a fence or hock it. I never got caught by the police, really. One time, though, they took me in 'cause I was the most probable suspect that did it, that stole some jewelry from this guy's house. His mother's jewelry at a party. But they didn't have any proof, so they had to let me go. They were right, though. I mean, I did it. I was the one. But I lied my way out of it. Blamed someone else. I ended up hocking the stuff at a pawnshop.

I sold drugs, too. I dealt cocaine and marijuana and 'ludes and all kinds of drugs. Before I'd start out I'd go steal a TV or something, you know, and I'd sell it for twenty bucks or whatever, and then I'd go get some drugs. My intention at that time would be to sell them, to make more money. But it always worked out that by the time I got 'em, ten minutes later they were all gone. I'd use 'em myself. So I was always getting deeper and deeper into it. You know what's amazing? If someone had told me before I ever started doing drugs that I'd end up stealing shit, I would never have believed it. Never in a million years. Not me. It didn't even feel like me anymore. I didn't feel like I was even alive. I was basically high all the time.

Then it got real serious—I started basing. It was about three months before my sixteenth birthday. I had to have it. I started getting into Valium; those I stole from my father. Then came PCP, and then 'ludes and reds and points [uppers]—all kinds of stuff. I never shot up heroin, but I took it in loads [capsule form]. Heroin was all right, you know. It was pretty good. But I got sick. That's why I didn't really like it. But after doing it a while, you know, it was all right.

Whatever I took I abused to the letter. I abused it as far as I could. As far as I could. I just kept taking more and more drugs, whatever I could get my hands on. More and more anything.

I ran away a few times. I couldn't stand it at home when I was using. I'd go to school to see if there were any doors open and sleep inside there somewhere, on the floor or whatever. Sometimes I could find a friend's house to sleep at—you know, in the garage or whatever. Usually I'd just stay in parks or someplace. Usually within five, seven days, I'd be back home again. I'd just come back, and my parents would be at work or something, and I'd just open the door and come in and go to sleep. I don't think they said anything to me ever about it. I know they were worried, I'm sure, but they didn't know how to deal with it. Sometimes they'd say something, you know, "Where were you?" They didn't usually. They knew if they asked too many questions I'd just leave again.

**Vic's drug usage increased as his senses of self-preservation and moderation declined. It was inevitable that one day he'd have to pay the price for his recklessness.**

I had started taking Valiums, like, about the end of my tenth grade summer. And then I didn't really take any more Valiums because I'd progressed into all the other drugs. But then I'd picked up a few more, like the winter of my sixteenth birthday. I woke up in the morning, like on a Thursday, and I took 'em through that whole day, and it was no problem, but I woke up Friday morning and took some, and I smoked some weed and drank some beer and did some cocaine and then took some more Valium. I started blacking out and forgetting how many I'd taken.

So I just kept taking them, 'cause I thought I needed them, or whatever. I wanted to get higher than I already was. And I kept taking 'em and taking 'em, and around noon I came home and sat down on the couch. I was watching TV. My mom came in and noticed something was wrong. She could see that I didn't look too well or anything. So she called the hospital and drove me to the emergency room. I guess I had overdosed. They pumped my stomach and gave me some stuff to drink, and I puked that back out, and then they sent me straight upstairs to their drug-rehabilitation center. The first few days, I was just laying down and was all—I felt like Jello. I can't really—everything's like a, in a fog. I burned my brain.

I was really pissed off at my mother for putting me there. I called her about every day and told her, you know, "Get me the hell out of here. I don't wanna be here, I don't need this, nothing's wrong, I don't have a problem." And she wouldn't, you know. She talked to the counselor. She wouldn't take me. She just left me in there.

**As angry as he was for being placed in a rehab program against his will, when the drug-induced haze began to lift, Vic began to realize that he was lucky just to be alive.**

Some of my friends are dead 'cause of drugs. Some people got shot for, like, burning people on drugs. You know, they sold bad drugs or got the drugs fronted and didn't pay for them. So, you know, they got killed—executed. Some of them weren't dealing with the right people. There's worse—there's bad and there's worse. These guys, the ones who got killed, got in with the worse people. I was a little more careful than they were. Or maybe I was just luckier. I bought from anybody I could get 'em from. Sometimes I could've gotten my butt shot off too, just by being in the wrong place at the wrong time. And I knew, you know, something was gonna happen someday. You know, I'd heard that this guy's got a whole bunch of drugs, or these other people are gonna come in and take 'em from him, you know. But I'd be there anyway to see what I could get after it was all over, you know. I was there when it was goin' on, and you know, they could've picked me up for one of his friends or whatever. I didn't really worry about it at all much. I guess I was stupid. Anyway, I was so drugged all the time, like walking around in a cloud, I couldn't think about anything other than scoring. There's a strong possibility that I would've been with a friend of mine the night that he got killed. I wasn't, and I was lucky.

I realized that there was something wrong in my life, to be running around with the kind of people I was. When I got in the hospital I realized, you know, all those feelings came back. 'Cause when you're in the hospital you don't get drugs. So the feelings start coming up. Everything that's been pushed down for so long.

**When he left the hospital, Vic had every good intention of staying clean. But he didn't for very long.**

I went in the hospital in early January, and I got out late May, and then when I got out I went right back home and stayed there for a couple months. But it just didn't work out with me and my parents, and also I had relapsed. I went out and started using again. I had not even thought about using that whole day or whole month, or whatever, you know, I was just gonna stay sober and stay away from all the friends. But one guy just came over and said, "Let's go somewhere, you know, let's just take a ride down to the beach and go surfing or something." So I said, all right, 'cause he was leavin' the next day to move out of the state. And we go down there, and then he just pulled out some lines, you know, cocaine, and I did it all up, and then after that, I said, "You know, shit, I fucked up." So I said, "As long as I fucked up, just go ahead and fuck it all." I went out that night and got drunk and smoked pot and did all this stuff. And the next morning I woke up, I really felt like shit.

When my mom find out, I got kicked out of the house. I guess my mom got fed up. We couldn't get along. I went straight to an AA meeting and shared about it and told everybody what happened. That night, right afterward, I got with some friends and got high, but when I woke up the next morning I said, "That's enough, that's enough." I went to another AA meeting and shared about it. This was the first time she ever kicked me out of the house. And so I made up my mind, this would be the last time. For a couple weeks I stayed with some sober friends. I didn't go back to any of my using friends 'cause I knew that was a bad deal. Then I convinced my mom to let me back in.

Me and my mom couldn't get along, though. There was just this conflict between us all the time. I think she kept thinkin' I was gonna start using again. I guess too much had gone down already. So she kicked me out of there. Just told me to get lost, get with my friends or something. I went straight to AA.

**One of the AA members gave Vic the name of a residential recovery house in his area.**

Now I'm real grateful. I've got a place to live, to sleep. I don't have to sleep on the street or in the parks. I came here, and my dad came to see me, you know, to sign all the papers and everything. Now I'm here and all the people here are great. Everyone wants everyone else to make it. We talk all the time. You get lots of time to think about stuff. Sometimes I think it'd be nice to be just a normal person, you know, not have to go through all this shit, but, but it happened, you know, it doesn't matter why it happened, it just happened, and now I've gotta learn to deal with it, learn to change.

Taking all those drugs when I did, there was a part of me that didn't grow. It got stunted. Now it's startin' to grow. My mental, emotional, physical, you know—that all got stunted. I felt sorry for myself a lot, like my parents were always on my back, like nobody likes me, you know, like I'm just a fuck-up or whatever. I didn't fit in with anybody. You know, I had a couple close using friends, but they were *using* friends, so it wasn't like there was any kind of bond between us.

I remember a long time ago in school they had a big assembly about drinking and driving, and a policeman came in there and said, "I'm not gonna tell you not to drink, but I'm telling you not to drink and drive." It didn't matter. He showed us pictures of bodies that'd been in accidents with drunk drivers, and they were all bloody and twisted up. But so what? No one thinks it's going to happen to them, just like I never thought I'd get to this point. You know, it's an old cliché, that you just can't say "Don't do it" to someone. I mean, they're gonna do it anyway. Even if I tell other kids not to do drugs 'cause of what happened to me, they're going to anyway if they want to. They'll say, "Oh yeah, that's just a bunch of baloney—you know, bullshit." It took me a long time to realize I needed help.

People think that everybody who's cool has to use drugs, and that is a whole bunch of BS. I used to believe that too, yeah. But now I can see where it's going to lead: The cool people are the ones who are not gonna be using drugs because they're the one who are gonna be alive. I think the people that are in the program here and now are gonna be the ones who make the future for the other kids. If we keep sharing our experiences and strength and hope, you know, then maybe some kids will start getting the message that drugs aren't really okay.

I remember a bum on the street came up and asked me for a cigarette, and he was drunk and was all feelin' down because he was tryin' to get sober and everything. I just talked to him and told him, "I know how you feel. It feels like shit being, you know, fucked up." But I said, "You don't have to do it, you know, you're drunk now but that doesn't mean you have to go get drunk tomorrow. You can stop. Go and get help." That's all it takes is just that one step. A guy has to get real bad before he can admit it. If my mother hadn't found me I might've just passed out for a few hours, woken up with a bad headache, and just gone right back out and did it again. That's if I lived. I was real lucky. There's most of those two years that I don't remember. They're just a blank.

# LORI

**"It felt so good not to feel bad."**

I started with pot, but after a while I didn't like it because it burned me out. So then I started drinking and it made me have fun; it made me happy. I was in the seventh grade when I started smoking pot. I didn't want to do it the first time. I guess it was peer pressure or whatever. My best friend asked me to do it, and I said no. Her brother was in the room and she goes, "We'll go in the back," 'cause I guess that would have made me feel more comfortable or something, and so I said, "No, no." 'Cause before that, when I was in sixth grade, it was like people would have joints all over my neighborhood. It was like gangs all the time, and they smoked pot, and I'd pick it up and I'd be all, "What the hell is this?" And so she said, "Okay, we'll do it in the back." And I said, "Okay, I'll do it," 'cause she kept saying it. And then I did it and it was like, it really didn't make me feel any kind of way. I felt, you know, like I'm bad. I think after the first two times I still didn't feel anything, and then after that it was like I was really hyper and really happy for like a half an hour and then anytime someone had pot or something I'd be like, "Let me have some, let me have some"—all the time. I don't know if I was addicted, it was just maybe 'cause I wanted to be accepted or have everybody think, "Oh, you know, she wants to do it." 'Cause, like, all my friends, they were stoners, you know, and they always had it. Always. I'm serious.

Towards the end of the eighth grade I was pretty much gettin' high all the time, but I wasn't liking it as much. Pot made me burn out. Like, I'd be hyper, happy for like a half an hour, and then for two hours I'd be sitting there like I was dead. Then when I got into the ninth grade I discovered JD—Jack Daniels. You only had to like drink a little bit. I'd go to bed or something, and then I'd wake up and I'd like taste it, that's all, nothing; it didn't give me headaches or nothing.

Lori, sixteen, was the daughter of a middle-class family. Her father, a hairstylist and photographer, moved the family each time he got a new job. Her mother, also a photographer, tried to pay close attention to the type of friends Lori chose, and she forced her to change them when she felt they were a bad influence. Drinking whiskey in the eighth grade was not the first experience Lori had with alcohol.

I drank when I was like eight or nine or something with my dad. We had a bottle of Heineken or something in the fridge and like my dad and my brother and sister were daring me to drink it. My mom wasn't there. And I'm like, "I'll drink it, you know." My dad was weird. It was like he was sadistic and stuff. He hurt me. He emotionally and physically molested all three of us—me, my brother, and sister from when we were little. I'm the youngest, my sister's about five years older, and my brother's three years older. Almost since she was born, when she was a baby, he first started like beating my sister up. He did, like, karate chops on the back of her neck, and when she would cry he'd stuff a blanket in her mouth. It's sad. I guess he did it 'cause she was getting more attention than he was or something.

I didn't even know that he used to beat me up when I was that young, but I have pictures of me when I was real little with bruises on my face. I have a bruise on my face and I didn't even notice it. I mean, I looked at this picture all through my life and I never noticed it, and I showed it to my counselor in the rehab and she goes, "What's that on your face?" And I'm like, "Oh, my God, there's a bruise on my face." It was weird. I mean, it's like, he beat me up every day of my life. We used to have a chalkboard that, if we did something wrong, he'd write how many whippings we'd get or how many times we're gonna get hit. And every day there'd be somebody's name on that chalkboard. He hit us every way: slug me in the stomach and tell me to close my eyes, that type of stuff.

He molested my sister. Like, he made her give him head since she was five till she was sixteen. I didn't have to do anything like that. He would take off all my clothes and laugh at me, you know, things like that; that's molesting, but it's not the same as my sister. My mom was there, but my mom was—it's like my mom was sick too. She wanted to get away from her family, so she married him real quick. They got married when he was nineteen and she was sixteen. And so she didn't have anywhere to turn, I guess. She was afraid of him. We were all afraid of him. He was like the king. Whatever he said, we did. When he burped, we said, "Excuse me." I'm serious, that's how it was. It's weird, 'cause he's not some macho guy. He's really a wimp. I mean, if you look at him, he's a wimp, but we were little, and he could, you know, fuck us up pretty bad.

I think what happened when he dared me to drink the beer was, he was trying to get my sister drunk. And I just happened to take it out, I guess to get attention or something, 'cause my sister got mass attention, 'cause she was the one gettin' molested all these years and we really didn't even know it. She seemed okay to me, 'cause I was living with her. But she never confided in me, I guess she was scared, and like sometimes I would kind of wonder, you know. I'd say, "Are you having an affair with my dad?" I was really protective of my mom, and I would really get angry, and she'd be like, "No, get the fuck away from me," and she'd get really defensive. And then, like one time, me and my brother caught her, and shit. They jumped when we walked in so it was kinda obvious. I remember I wrote my mom a note, and she didn't believe me.

But that time when we were drinking, he took out all this wine and stuff and liquor out of the cupboard, and he's all like trying to make my sister drink it, so that he can get her drunk. And then, I guess, I just took that beer and I go, "I think I'm gonna down this. How much will you guys give me?" And they're all, "We'll give you this much." So then I drank it all. And I was like, hmm . . . I was all proud of myself, you know. I don't know why I didn't just start drinking then. It was just like, something that we didn't do, you know. Nobody in my family drank, 'cause my dad had ulcers. Nobody did drugs, either. I think maybe the feeling of having that drink might of been in my subconscious mind when I first got high. I think I just realized it when I wrote down that my dad was trying to get my sister drunk, and I gave the note to my mom. So I think that's when I realized it. But she didn't believe me.

I drank with my best friend. Her name's Connie. We used to have guys come into the girls' bathroom at school and we'd all drink. There was no narcs then; well, they didn't come in the bathrooms. We could just smoke in there and not even worry about anybody. At that point, we were drinking or gettin' high, like maybe, let's see—it was always on the weekends, 'cause I only got to go out one day; I only got to be out of the house, except for school, on Saturdays, from eleven to four. I couldn't go out at night, or on Sundays. My parents wouldn't let me. They wanted me around all the time. And that's why I started ditchin'. Me and my mom used to hit each other. We hit the fuck out of each other. I'm serious. Because of that and other shit. Just 'cause of stupid things. We'd get in arguments all the time—me and my mom, me and my brother, me and my sister, me and my dad. I have all these scars on my face—you have to look close to see them now—from all the fighting.

**When Lori was in the seventh grade, she finally convinced her mother that her father had been incredibly abusive. After**

a number of failed attempts at separation, her mother divorced him and was married soon thereafter to her employer.

She was like living with this guy right after the divorce. She was seeing him before we left my dad. And that was her boss. It was my dad and her boss. And so my mom married him 'cause they got to be real good friends. He had kids too. See, he got a divorce with his wife, 'cause his wife had an abortion without telling him. His kids hate us, 'cause they feel that we took him away from them. Anyway, he hit me too. He said I instigated him or something. Like I was—I wanted attention. I was a people-pleaser, you know? Act real stupid and people would laugh, and then that would make me happy.

The first time he hit me, they weren't even married yet. I was like playing around. I put my blanket over him and stuff, and he was acting along, you know, like putting the blanket over his head and he was going, "Ooh." And then I got in the back of him 'cause he put the blanket over me, and I think I was holding him in a head lock or something, but I don't think I was holding him tight. And then he flipped me over his head, hard, and I was like, "Whoa," you know, 'cause I thought we were playing. And I just like fully went boom on the ground. I was like, "Fucking asshole!" I just went off. I started yelling at him and everything. And my mom started yelling at me, you know, "Don't talk to my boyfriend this way." And I was like, "God, what an asshole," and he got really pissed, and he hit me for it. He did it right in front of my mom, and she just didn't say anything to him. She just like got mad at me.

The situation improved, Lori said, once the entire family began seeing a psychiatrist. But since that didn't occur until years later, the years in between were equally perilous, and Lori continued to drink and smoke pot to help alleviate the pain. She said, though, that even at his worst, her stepfather was much preferable to her real father. "It's like anybody really was better than him. Even a rapist. 'Cause my dad wasn't really worth a shit."

The summer after eighth grade, oh God, that was the worst summer. They told me I had to stay home every day and that I couldn't watch TV till four o'clock, couldn't talk on the phone till six-thirty, and during that time, the whole time I had to do something constructive like read a newspaper and write a report on it. It was like, just to make myself smarter. See, my stepdad had a straight-A-student daughter, you know, and so like he was trying to make us better, like pointing out, "All you have to do is fix this and you'll be perfect." We'd fix that and then it would be, "All you have to do is fix this," and on and on. And we'd have to work on, like, revenge and shit like that, like guilt trips; we'd work on all these things, 'cause we were going to the child guidance clinic. And they gave us a book on all this shit, and it used to piss me off so bad. And I couldn't go out, so I started sneaking out at night, at midnight, and go knocking on my friends' windows. We'd like go out and party sometimes, or we'd just walk around and talk, and smoke our cigarettes. But I mean, it was fun.

In ninth grade, that's when I really started hanging around with guys a lot. There was only two girls in the whole crowd, and there was a lot of guys. Mass attention. I couldn't go to parties, 'cause I still wasn't allowed out of the house. I still only had those five hours on Saturday. So what I did in tenth grade was, I started ditching. At first a little, and I got away with it, so then a lot. During the summer, I ran away for two weeks and got high every day. My parents called the police. They were looking for me.

Tenth grade was worse. All I did was smoke pot and drink. It really got to every day. I ditched every day. But I stopped smoking pot in December of tenth grade, 'cause

I'd burned out too much. And all I did was drink. A bunch of us would ditch and get beer and hang out in this big concrete wash—it was like a big bunker sort of thing. We'd go on a beer run. We'd go in a van and we'd go in a store and steal a case and we'd drive off. The guys would do it. You just take it and then, when they're not looking, I guess you just run out. The guys'd go in the van and we'd drive off down the alley, and we'd hang out all day and drink beer. I always got at least four. My stepdad would look at me funny sometimes when I got home, and my brother was always going, "Lori smokes pot." I'm like, "No I don't, no I don't." 'Cause he went to school with me and he saw me at school and he saw the people I hung around with, you know, and I was—I had big resentments against him. He always said, "Well, you're loaded. You're fucked up, huh?" And I was like, "No." The times when I wasn't, you know, pissed me off.

Still in the tenth grade, Lori was arrested when she and her girlfriend visited another high school during school hours to meet other people they knew.

I wanted to get drunk and go in there and visit everybody. We hitchhiked. This guy bought us beer and then we went there. I was just gonna go in there and say, "Hi, what's up?" I was just loaded, and I felt like visiting them. We didn't even get a chance to go in the school, and the narcs caught us over where we were at, across the street. There's a church and there were steps, and we were sitting on the steps. And they saw us drinking on the steps. I guess that wasn't too smart, but see, I thought alcohol was good—better than pot, because pot was illegal and you're allowed to drink alcohol when you're twenty-one; I thought it was okay. I mean, I would walk around with a beer and not even worry about it. I'm serious. That was my way of justifying it: pot's illegal, this isn't.

So anyway, they took us down to the police station, and then they called my mom and everything, and I was being really rude, 'cause I was buzzed. I was all like, "Keep your fucking hands off me," that kind of thing. And like they handcuffed me and I took my hands out of the handcuffs. I was like, "Ha, look at this." I pulled 'em out. They didn't tighten 'em enough. It was funny. So my mom came down and afterwards she said, "I don't know if I'm gonna come get you," so I was like, fuck, you know, and then after that, I went back to school and everything. I mean, I tried to go back to school. I hadn't been there in a long time. Right when I came back, that day I had to go to the office and they kicked me out 'cause of the thing with the cops—plus they'd caught me smoking twice before, so I guess that was the last straw.

Lori enrolled in another school in the same school district.

I was still getting loaded and ditching from the new school, you know, meeting my old friends at the wash and drinking. And then I got suspended for being drunk on campus. I got caught. I didn't get arrested, but my punishment was getting put in this detox place, a rehab. My mom did it. She made me get a urinalysis, and then they told her that I was probably on drugs a lot. I told her that I'd try to keep straight, and they said I had to come there every day. But when I got there I ran away again and went and got loaded. They busted me, though. The way they did it was, I told my ex-boyfriend to come to the place. I go, "It's really cool, you'll like it." And I ran away the day before he was supposed to start, you know, and like I told him I was getting loaded. I stayed all over. I was staying in another ex-boyfriend's van, and I was staying with my best friend's boyfriend and her, 'cause she ran away too. She's still running away, and I'm the one who introduced drugs to her, and she's doing heroin now, and she's way fucked up. And it's like, it just trips me out, because I didn't get that far, you know, and I'm thankful for that.

Brian told my counselor that I was getting loaded, and I was sitting there lying, saying I wasn't. I told him I was, he said, and I said I wasn't. Drugs made me a liar. Ever since I was with my dad I was a liar anyways, though, 'cause I had to lie in order to not get hit. And so I'm sitting there and I'm like, "I didn't get loaded," and they knew already I did. I lied to everybody except my friends, 'cause my friends were my life. It was like I was really like against teachers and shit like that. Any kind of authority. If it hadn't been for my friends . . . I was at the point when I got to the rehab that I wanted to kill myself. I was writing all these poems and shit, and just really, I was real bad. See, when all this shit falls on you, when you get caught for all this shit, you feel really bad and you're just like you don't think you're gonna live another day without getting in trouble or feeling really shitty. And I hated to feel bad. It's like, right now, I'm at the point where someone could say to me, "I don't like this about you," and I'll feel like, "Oh, God, they don't like this about me, what am I gonna do?" It's like, everything hurts my feelings where I'm at right now. That's what happens when you stop drinking. I would hide it with alcohol—at least for then, you know? I'd get kind of numb.

**Lori said she thought she had lost the ability to have fun without getting loaded in some way. She couldn't even have straight friends.**

I had a boyfriend that was sober. I mean, sort of. See, I only saw him on the weekends, and then 'cause of me, he started drinking; I got him drinking. 'Cause it was like, "I want to have fun. What are we gonna do?" What else are you supposed to do? See, 'cause when you ditch there's not much you can do, 'cause there's, like, these truant guys all over, and you can't go anywhere. We went to the park sometimes when I ran away, we got drunk there. But it was like we were scared all the time, so we figured we'd go to the wash and get drunk. It was kind of like out where nobody was, and that was our way of having fun, and that's the only way I thought that you could have fun after a while—doing that like a lot.

Before I started drinking I knew how to have fun without being loaded, but I totally forgot about it. Anyway, it didn't matter 'cause I only had a few hours a week to fuck around with my friends. Fuck, even in the summer—it was worse in the summer. My stepdad wanted us always in the house. He started taking power, like saying, "Well, these kids, they're just fucking around, they're not doing anything good for themselves." So we had to stay in the house and all this shit. Every once in a while we'd get to go to the public pool and swim there for a day or something. Even my sister, she was eighteen too, and she still had to. Ever since she was born—when she was born to sixteen she didn't get to go out. It was like, who cares about summer? It was worse 'cause I had to stay home with my dad every fuckin' day. We had to stay home and clean house—fun, you know? It's like, "Oh, no, summer!"

**From a sober perspective now, Lori has spent a lot of time analyzing and dissecting her past behavior. Even though she had a multitude of factors which might be considered responsible for her alcohol and drug addiction, she says she refuses to blame anyone but herself.**

I did all the things that all drug addicts do. Like vandalizing shit. I thought I was so tough. I put on this image that I was real tough shit. I'd dress like a guy, wore my Levis and my sneakers, and my t-shirt; I'd dress totally like a guy. I'd be like, you know, like I'd wanna fight anyone who dresses the way I do now—you know, like a girl, like feminine. I got in lots of fights. Anybody that fucked with me. I had a real attitude when I was loaded, but even when I wasn't. Even when I was living with my dad, it's like anybody that would say anything bad about me or anything, if they would hurt my feelings, and call me stupid—'cause my dad called me stupid a lot—I'd beat on 'em. Then I didn't understand why. It was just like I thought everybody's family was like my family, everybody got beat up, everybody got called stupid and ugly and da-da-da-da. And everybody got laughed at when they were naked or whatever. And so it was like when people would do that, it would hurt my feelings. So if somebody hurt my feelings I'd just like, fully go off on 'em. But it was like I would always wait for them to hit me first, 'cause I thought I wouldn't get busted. Even now, I still hit guys sometimes. But I try not to 'cause it's not good. Sometimes when I get real mad I hit my boyfriend, but not that often.

Lori explained that she never did any other drugs than marijuana and alcohol. She didn't believe they were as addicting as cocaine, heroin, and barbiturates. "But," she said, "I know I would've kept going and probably done all that other shit, 'cause I was getting to the point where I wanted to commit suicide."

When I first got into rehab, I must've run away and used and lied about it eight times. I'd just take off and get high and say I wasn't. But finally, once I saw how people were having fun when they were sober, it made me feel better about it, and so I tried it. I got nine months sober now. I used to have weird ideas about sober people. All the sober people at school I knew were like into books—you know, nerdy kind of people. It's like I can really remember myself saying to my boyfriend, "Oh, let's have fun, let's go get somebody to get beer." We'd bum money outside of 7-Eleven stores. We'd get somebody that walked up into 7-Eleven. It felt so good not to feel bad, but I didn't know there was anything wrong with me at the time. I didn't know that I felt bad, I just thought that was the way I was—the way everyone was.

Now when I see all my old friends—'cause I try to avoid everyone I used to hang with when I was drinking—they come up to me, "Lori, why don't you party anymore? You too good for us?" And stuff like that. I'm like, "Fuck you, get away," and they just get all mad. They just don't understand. Some people do. Some people do, but some people don't.

**Asked why she, too, didn't end up as a hard-core heroin addict, like her friend whom she introduced to drugs, Lori said she credits her mother for forcing her back into a rehab program.**

I probably would be real bad, you know. I mean, I don't like looking at my mom as, like, you know, "You're a bitch," or anything anymore. I mean, if I'm mad at her or something, I might really cop an attitude and be real mad at her. I know she made a bunch of mistakes, but it's kinda like, I don't know. I'm in denial with my mom right now. It's kinda like, I don't want to say my mom is bad. I mean, I still love my dad too, you know, and he did real weird stuff. My mom's really sweet, see. She's getting better right now. She's going to all these things— how-to-be-good-parent stuff—and she reads all these books to find out how kids are and stuff. And it's like she's a really sweet person. It's just that my dad fucked her up. My dad beat her up too, and he did a whole bunch of shit to her as much as he did to us.

# J.D.

**"What people think is that there's an age group or a race group or whatever, but it hits everybody and anybody it wants to, and that's it. There's no restrictions. It's not prejudiced whatsoever. And so you just never know."**

Let's see, I was about thirteen or fourteen when I started drinkin' a little beer, smokin' a little pot—you know, with my friends, socially, peer-pressure kind of stuff. I know for sure I was fourteen when I was introduced to cocaine. It was by an older friend. I wasn't one of those type of people that, you know, didn't like it the first time. I hear a lot of people don't get high the first time or don't like it. But I liked it immediately. I got high and liked it and did it again. I guess that was the beginning of my downfall.

I was very upset when I went into the hospital and found out that I couldn't drink anymore. I thought the program was about being abstinent from all mind-altering substances—period. And you know, at first I didn't understand why, and now I do, because for one thing I did abuse alcohol. I didn't realize it, but I did drink on a daily basis. You name it, I drank it. From beer to whiskey. I didn't always feel I abused it, though, because it didn't usually—at first it didn't interfere with things. The thing was, you know, when I used coke I would drink to come down. That's a kind of common cycle. Before that, for a while I took Quaaludes, but they weren't as easily available—alcohol was much much easier to get.

J.D. was twenty-one when he finally entered a drug-and-alcohol-rehabilitation program. In the previous seven or eight years, he had abused almost every kind of mind-altering drug: LSD, amphetamines, marijuana, alcohol, psilocybin mushrooms, cocaine, barbiturates, heroin. He came from a middle class home; he lived with his mother following his parents' divorce when he was eight. He saw his father, who remarried and moved several miles away, at most every few weeks.

I worked at this market, where it was easy to steal alcohol. I guess I was about sixteen. At first I got the job at the market in order just to have some money, some extra money, 'cause I was living with my mom, and she took care of everything—clothes and food and all that stuff. After my parents got divorced, my mom had to kind of struggle, she had to work, to put my brother and me through private schools and all that, but I had what I needed. I certainly wasn't hurting. I went to good schools, had clothes, you know, was given a car when I was sixteen, etcetera. Anyway, after a while, I started needing more money for liquor and drugs than I could get by working. So I stole the stuff; that's the reason I stayed at the job. It was kind of fun, because my friends would come over and I'd supply all the liquor and we'd party, you know, and that made me feel like the big man. I was living at home, but I had a room outside that's all mine because I'm a musician, I play the drums. They were loud, and so we had a den out there. I moved out there when I went into high school, you know, so I could play, so the band could come over.

I always felt like I was close to my mom, but when I got really heavy into the drug scene, we started fighting a lot. I think she knew I was using. I came to her when I was about, I don't know, fifteen or so. And I told her that I wanted to smoke pot. And at the time, my stepfather, the guy that she was livin' with, that was livin' with us, smoked pot. So what she decided was, instead of having me run out on the streets and doin' it out there where I could get in a lot of trouble, she said it would be okay if I just did it at home—as long as it didn't interfere with my schoolwork. You know, if I never drank and drove, that kind of thing.

You know, I've told a couple people about that since, and they said how hip they thought she was. But the thing is, since I've been in this program I've realized how manipulative that was of me to do. In a way, I used the guilt that she had over the divorce to get what I wanted. I knew I was manipulating her, you know, by telling her that I wanted to use drugs. That kind of put her on the spot, because she could say no, but then she'd know I'd go out on the streets and use it anyway. And I knew she wouldn't throw me out, 'cause I knew how much she loved me. So in a way that was a big manipulation to be able to get to use around my home. By telling her, trying to make it look like I'm really being honest—"Mom, here I am, I'm using drugs, but I'm gonna be mellow, just do it in the house, you know." You know that's a manipulation. Just in a general way, when I wanted something I would just ask for it, and I would usually get it. And I'd use that to my advantage.

Later on, as I got older, around seventeen, she realized that she couldn't have given me everything anyway or whatever. She was getting upset and would threaten to throw me out, that kinda thing. I guess she got tired of it, the manipulation, but deep down I knew she never would throw me out. She would threaten me, but I knew it would never happen. Even in my late stages of using, when I was such a wreck, stealing and the whole thing, she never threw me out. And I knew she wouldn't. So I used that to my advantage, to stay home and get my bills paid and spend all my paychecks on drugs and things—rather than having to pay rent. If I was out on my own, I'd have to pay my lawyer, and that was likely to slow me down at least, if it didn't stop me entirely. You know, I had it made. Until I went into the hospital three months ago, I'd lived at home all my life. Being here is, like, my first time out on my own. It really upset her when I told her in the hospital that I'm gonna go into a recovery home. She had no idea how bad things had gotten. She really wanted me to come back home.

When J.D. finally checked himself into a rehab program, he had already come close to death several times. Until the very end, those close brushes only seemed exciting; when he was using, he had almost no will to live.

It's funny, you know. It's really amazing that I did eventually care enough to get into a program. I came close to death five times. In a way, I think I might have wanted to die. But I know I didn't really care. I didn't feel like there was anything to live for. Especially around the end, because I did start realizing that I was addicted, and I had no respect for myself or anyone. I was real ashamed. But even earlier, it was like I didn't care. I mean, I was fourteen years old when I had my first seizure, and it wasn't like I was suicidal or anything like that, but it was, I think, the thrill, the danger, knowing afterward that I'd come real close to dying.

The guy that introduced me to coke was real into freebasing. What happened was, I was sitting on a chair and I took a hit, and the next thing I know I'm wakin' up on the floor in the hallway in the next room, and I'm looking up at the ceiling just spinning, and I'm gettin up and my friend's just cryin', and he's got blood on his hands. And I couldn't figure out what the hell was goin' on, and he's tellin' me, "Just sit down and I'll tell you, just sit down." So then he told me: I was sitting in a chair and I started shaking after I took a hit. I went into convulsions. And I'm bouncing, and I flipped off the chair, and I'm on the ground, and I'm still floppin' around. And what he was doin', the reason his hand was bloody, was 'cause he was sticking his fingers in my mouth to keep me from swallowing my tongue, and I was biting on him, you know, from the seizure, and I was chomping on his hands. The lucky thing was, the house that we were at, that we were partying at, there just happened to be this guy who knew CPR [cardio-pulmonary resuscitation]. Well, he wasn't there right at the beginning, but he comes running in with a gun, you know, waving the gun around, and says he thought somebody was robbing the place. He had a lot of coke around. Mind you, this is all what they told me later; I was unconscious all this time. Well, then he realized what was goin' on, and he dropped the gun, and—I guess right before he came in, I had just completely stopped breathing. They said I wasn't breathing, and they didn't get a heartbeat, nothin'. And he did CPR on me. I don't know how long I was out of it, I'm sure it wasn't as long as it probably seemed to them. But the crazy thing is, I was ready to hit the pipe again right after I came to. You know, I don't think it was really suicidal or anything, I never really believed that it could happen—that I could die.

On through the years I've had four more seizures. The last time was just a few months ago, in my room. In fact, I've had most of 'em in the last few months that I was using. Always after freebasing. One time it was in front of my brother. My friends had to call the ambulance, and I came to just as the ambulance got there. I must've been out for a little while, 'cause I got up and walked outside my door and the ambulance was pullin' up in front of the house. They took me to the hospital and checked me out and then sent me home. But I had a couple of seizures when I was alone, too. I'd wake up and my drum set would be knocked over, bruises all over me from where I was falling on stuff and hitting the ground. And you know, I didn't stop. I did it again. It didn't bother me somehow. I don't know why, I think it was just the progression of the disease. I was so addicted that I had to get my high. Live or die, it didn't matter.

You know, I guess I was addicted more to living on the edge than the drugs themselves. Well, maybe that's true. I just thought of that just now, 'cause I'm thinking about this time I got mixed up with a guy and robbed a bank. He'd been doin' it for a while, and we were kind of hangin' out and everything, so I finally decided to do it myself. And I got caught. The first time I ever did it. You know, I owed people money for drugs, and I had to get more drugs, so I definitely needed the money. But it was the thrill again, the excitement, the danger. I didn't want to get killed—at least, not when I was straight. But when I was using the drugs I didn't care whether I lived or died kinda thing. I didn't feel anything, I was high, and I figured if I went out, well, I'm high anyway—that kind of thing. As long as I had the high, the world was fine. I knew I could have a seizure and die, but so what?

I was high when I robbed that bank. I don't know how, but by the grace of God I happened to get off on probation. I just happened to have a clean record and had a good lawyer, and the whole thing was reduced to robbery rather than armed robbery. What I did was, I passed the teller a note. I went to a certain bank where there's no security, and it just—you know, I knew how to do it from watching on TV and in the movies. I wasn't armed, and so I somehow got off on five years' probation. Getting shot in a robbery woulda been dramatic, but I don't think I could've shot at someone myself, that's what I'm tryin' to say. Anyway, it all scared me so much that I didn't use for about a year, year and a half. Oh, maybe I drank a little bit, smoked a little pot.

Somewhere along the line I started up again, about a year, year and a half later, and I used all sorts of shit for about a month or two. I could see it happenin' again, the old patterns, and amazingly enough, it scared me enough, and I said, "No, I'm not gonna do it." And I stopped and started working out, and I started running, and I got really into my health, which I'd always been off and on with the exception of the drugs. It's really kind of weird. It's like it's Jekyll and Hyde. When I'm not on cocaine, I watch what I eat, I watch what I drink. Maybe drink a little bit of beer, maybe smoke a joint, you know, but not overdo anything. But man, I get on that cocaine and it's a totally different thing. I mean, it's like I don't care about anything or anybody. I become like a kind of thief—steal from my own mother to get it, and that's about as low as you can get. I didn't really become violent. I was very mellow. I've always been a very mellow guy. But after I've drunk I've gotten violent before. I've picked fights with huge bouncers in clubs. I'd find out later; I'd come back the next day and my friends would show me this guy who's like six feet two that I'd chosen off. You know, I mean, I'm not very big, and, I mean, look at this guy, built like a brick shithouse, and I'm a jerk pickin' a fight with him 'cause I was drunk.

After two or three months of excessive drug use following that year and a half of sobriety, J.D. met a girl and fell in love. For a while, he says, she became his drug.

I was going to this trade school to get a certificate in computer programming, and that's where I met Debi; she worked there. She was just a gorgeous girl. I was just totally infatuated with her, and the drugs just didn't even enter my mind. Everything was just goin' hunky-dory. Then I started going to a university for a while to study engineering, and things just started fallin' apart. I couldn't make the grades, and it wasn't because I was using, and that's what really got me down. If I could at least blame it on using, you know, I woulda had an out, but I didn't. I just couldn't hack it. I've always been able to do anything I put my mind to, and that was a real mindblower. I really got blown out by that, that I could not do it.

So that kinda fell apart, and I started working, and somewhere along the line I took a snort of coke. I think I was at a dance with Debi, in fact, and one thing led to another, and pretty soon, you know, with me bombin' out in school, we weren't gettin' along. Part of it was probably because I was using a little bit—but not a lot, using here and there; it probably changed my own temperament. I was probably getting a little disinterested. Then I started to go and use the drugs again, and that meant we weren't spending as much time together. All this was happening all at once, and then she just came to me and said that she wanted to break up, that she wanted to go out with other guys. That just blew me away. She was a really beautiful girl. She was gorgeous. That was like the last-straw, I-couldn't-take-any-more kinda thing, and I just said, "Well, I don't have to deal with this, I can just go get high." It was a pretty conscious decision. I was even kinda shocked myself that I said that, 'cause I'm not usually like that. You know, I tried to play it off in front of everybody, that it was no big deal, but it really was a big deal to me, it really blew me out of the water. I just wasn't ready for it. So I said, "I'm just gonna get high, and everything's gonna be cool."

The next thing I know, I'm stealing from my work to get money to buy drugs. I was working at a restaurant as a host, and I used to tap the till. Then I became a waiter, and I would get money through the checks—you know, make-out-on-change kind of thing. I didn't really steal the alcohol from the restaurant, but for about six weeks before I was fired, I was a bartender and I would drink once in a while on the job, which wasn't cool. But that was kinda rare. I was mostly into just getting the money and leaving and doing coke. At that point, I was not drinking or even smoking pot, which was like a daily thing for me for a few years before that. Now, it was the cocaine was all I wanted, and I didn't even care about taking downs or drinking to come down from it. I would open a beer, and it would be sittin' there all night, and I wouldn't drink it. I mean, it was like just cocaine was all I wanted; it was all I needed.

It was pretty scary because I could see myself being a junkie. I mean, it was like a fix. I'd get my money, I'd leave work, I'd go straight by the rock house, come home, and I couldn't get to that pipe fast enough. I hit it, and then it was like, "Aah, now I'm okay." And a couple of times it hit me, "Wow, this is something out of the movies, just like a heroin addict or somethin'." It started becoming a thing where I was up three and four days. I'd just keep using around the clock: go to work to get more money to use—just go around the clock. I wouldn't sleep for three or four days. Then I'd finally pass out for a day or two when I had a day off.

I looked terrible. I lost about twenty-five pounds; I weighed about a hundred and twenty pounds. Some of my friends, the ones that cared, would ask me about it and try to tell me, "You know, why are you doing this to yourself?" Of course, I denied it: "Oh, I'm not doin' that." At this point I was doing the drugs by myself. I became selfish, and I wanted it all for me. I also think deep down that I was ashamed, so it was easier to not—to not see them. That way I didn't have to deal with them either. I had this one friend of mine that's been with me like two or three times when I've had a seizure, and it just scares the hell out of him. He doesn't want to be around me. So I was losing friends rapidly. I lost respect for them, I called them late, three in the morning, calling them and their folks with bullshit stories to get money, like an emergency for the car or something—you know, just to get more drugs. And it was obvious, I mean, it was blatant what I was doing. I didn't realize it, but it was, and I just—you know, I was losin' them, and I didn't care about that either. Just as long as I had my coke.

At that point, I could see that I was an addict. I mean, it was obvious. This whole thing went on like this every night for a couple months at least. I based in the bathroom at work, too, to get through until that night till I had money to leave and score more dope. Amazingly enough, I did my job well enough at work, but then again, it was noticeable that I was wasted. I mean, not wasted like I was drunk. See, on coke it wasn't like I was drunk where I was dropping plates and things, but I would shake, you know, like 'round the end of the night if I had none, I'd get real tired and be blinkin' my eyes like I was gonna pass out. People could see something was goin' on, I mean, it was just so obvious. When I first got the job, I really took care of myself. I was really into health and the whole thing, and I looked pretty good and blah blah. So when that finally fell apart . . .

J.D. was forced to leave his job when the restaurant manager, who had been somewhat of a friend, caught him stealing from the cash register. But rather than call the police, he gave J.D. a choice: Either he could sign a confession or a resignation. Obviously, he chose the latter.

He realized that I had a problem. I'd come to him once before and said I wanted to get insurance and I wanna take care of this problem, that I'd been doin' a lot of dope and I wanted to get into a detox. I mean, that's how close we were. And I never pursued and got the insurance together; I just kept using. I just got heavier and heavier and heavier, and finally I got caught. So I had no job, no friends, no nothing. I was stealing from my mother, stealing money and things out of her purse to get dope. That's got to be the lowest thing I ever did. You know, I never went and killed anybody for it or anything like that. If I had to sell something out of my room—you know, hock it—I'd do that too. I also borrowed money, but it didn't take long to run out of people to borrow from, 'cause I naturally never paid it back. I would do everything I could, you know, without going too far. I mean, I was on probation, and if I could go the whole five years without getting in trouble with the law again, then they'd seal the records from the robbery.

That scared me. I was in total lack of control. Absolutely no control. Cocaine controlled me, I didn't control it. And I looked in the mirror—I looked awful. Just, I really looked at myself. I looked dead. Before, people were telling me the same thing, but I really wouldn't believe it. And it was just such a cycle. It was just a terrible feeling. I felt so low. No friends, no anything. My family noticed it. Even some of my distant relatives who hadn't seen me in a while, they saw me and just thought I looked terrible. And it was just embarrassing, the whole thing. I was ashamed.

**While undergoing treatment, J.D. spent a lot of time trying to find explanations for his behavior.**

I don't think I ever blamed my parents for getting divorced. I never blamed my problems on their divorce. But, you know, I don't think I could have gotten away with some of the shit I did if I'd been living with my dad. But I'm just an obsessive person. You know, I'm obsessed with everything. I'm obsessed with sports, with school, with girlfriends, with music, with different things at different times—and it just happened to be the drugs. When I tried them, they just took me under. I tried them, I liked them, and I liked the feeling, I liked the feeling of being high, the euphoria. I loved to go to amusement parks and take acid you know, and I just—I liked experimenting. It seemed like anything I tried I liked.

When I was a kid they showed us these movies about drug addicts. And I remember thinking how weird that was to be. They showed these movies with heroin addicts with needles sticking out of their arms, and it was real dramatic. And the thing is, heroin is still the drug I'm still most afraid of. But from what I've heard, what the psychiatrist from my hospital told me, freebasing with cocaine is more addictive than anything. Including heroin. It's amazing how fast you can get addicted, you know. You can use it a month and be an addict. You know, like one week you'll do a gram, two weeks you'll be doin' two grams, three weeks you'll do three or four, and it just doubles and triples and quadruples just like that. Your tolerance goes up real quick. And the thing is, with cocaine, it's a big rush, and it's a very high euphoric feeling, but it only lasts a very very short time—two minutes, ten minutes. Maybe at first it lasts longer, maybe thirty, but as you do it more it gets down quicker, and you come down harder, and it's a very depressing feeling coming down. It's a terrible feeling coming down. So you have to get more to get back up there. That's why I kept stealing and things, 'cause I didn't want to come down. I never wanted to come down.

Like I already said, at the end there, I was running away from the pain of my relationship with Debi, but in a way I'd been running away all along from something. At first—I'm not going to deny it—I liked it; I was having a good time on 'em. But I didn't realize what it would make me do eventually. See, what happens is, eventually it doesn't do what it's supposed to do anymore; you can't just use it once, get a great high, and leave it alone. The tolerance is too high, and it just doesn't work for you. To me, it was like there's no way I could be an alcoholic or an addict. I mean, here I am going through a private prep school, you know, and there's kids dropping out of high school left and right. They were the ones, they were the drug addicts and alcoholics, not me. To me, an alcoholic is a Skid Row bum. I didn't have any idea that that was only one percent of the alcoholics out there. And I kept jobs. I always managed to hold a job, you know. If I put my mind to something, I could do it. The drugs were just like things that I did on the side. And until the end, they didn't seem to dominate me—but the end came real quick, and then it was just twenty-four hours a day.

Those seven or eight years that J.D. used drugs—a period in which most young people are are going through tremendous changes physically, emotionally, and intellectually—are now just a distant blur of memories; who, what, when, where, how, and especially why are disjointed and have no common thread in his mind.

When you're a kid, you want to be one thing one minute and something else the next. There was never anything I ever really wanted to be like a doctor or a lawyer, something that I wanted real badly. Well, I did always want to go to college. I went to a junior college for a semester, and I barely got through it, so when the second semester started I just dropped out. I'm trying to think why. I think I was just disinterested at the time. I don't really remember if it was drugs or what. You know, a lot of it's hazy, off-and-on stuff. Like I said, I would use for a while, stop for a while, use for a while, stop for a while . . .

I don't remember some of the reasons why I did things. You know, I kinda had dreams of getting my own little apartment and leaving, 'cause at this point I was gettin' older and I couldn't get along with my mother too well. I just felt like it was time to get a good job and leave. Then what happened was, I ended up going to computer-programming school. But see, my idea was to get a college degree, then fall back on that kind of thing. And that didn't work out, and instead of just going back and getting right back into the computer thing, I just started sliding all the way out; I just started using instead.

That was another thing, I always wanted something more. I always had to have more. I always set very high goals for myself, and of course didn't reach 'em, so depression, etcetera, always set in. And today I'm learning that material things aren't that big of a deal. You know, society puts on you that you gotta have money, you gotta be successful, you gotta have a house, and blah-blah. So I got wrapped up into that. I thought everything had to be successful. I had to be successful. I had to be an engineer because my dad was an engineer. I realize now that that's not true, that I never really wanted to be an engineer. I only tried it because he was, and he's great at it. Ever since I was a little kid I was very competitive—competing for grades, competing on the playground, competing at home. The funny thing is, I guess I'm learning, is that when I took drugs they made me not compete very well; I couldn't because they fucked me up so much. It's probably because I was never happy with myself.

**What about peer pressure?**

That's another thing. I hung out with older guys and they did it, and so I thought it was cool. I think that's a big thing. Even though maybe they wouldn't tell me, "Hey, you know, you gotta do this, you know, or we're not gonna like you," in a way that's how it feels. You think, "Well, I could be accepted if I drink like them, and if I learn to down beers." The whole thing: learn to drink like they drink, and learn to use like they use. And then, of course, being such an obsessive person myself it didn't take me long to just take it on my own anyway, where I just did it on my own whether they did or not. You know, I didn't have a lot of friends my age. I hung out with older guys most of the time, with the exception of my school buddies or my brother's friends. But I didn't really hang out with them. I liked hanging out with the older crowd. For one thing, I wasn't real popular in school. I was kind of small, and I wasn't really a great athlete—even though I wanted to be. Older friends that were more mature, you know, they accepted me for who I was, and then I partied with 'em. They didn't care that I wasn't a star football player or whatever. High school can get very nasty that way, in making you feel like you're a leper or something if you're not like everyone else.

What you don't realize until you get older is that it's not everyone else making you feel that way—it's you feeling like that yourself. They probably would have accepted me any way I was as long as I accepted myself; I'm really realizing that today. I always tried to be what everybody else wanted me to be. And today I'm just me, and you can accept it and take it or you don't have to and you can leave it and it doesn't bother me. A few months ago, it would've shook me up: "He doesn't like me 'cause of why? Well, maybe I better do that, then—so he'll like me. Or she'll like me." You know, especially with girls, I always tried to please them and do everything that I thought they wanted me to do. And I don't do that now. I mean, sometimes I'll catch myself doing that. That's what's really funny. When you're a kid, especially in high school, you think you gotta drink or use to be accepted. But people just don't care, you know, and I really don't care if they don't like it if I don't drink myself, see, 'cause I care about myself, and I know I'm one drink or one fix, I'm one hit away from right where I'm used to be. I can be an addict tomorrow. I can't just have it. I can never drink the way I drank before. I can never use the way I used at first. I just can't do it like other people. That's the way it is.

Everybody thinks it's cool to use; for me now, it's cool not to use. It was impossible to see that when I was younger, because you want to get accepted. But if anybody asked me, if you told me, you know, I was gonna end up here, I woulda never believed you. What happens is, the high burns out, you see, 'cause once you get dependent on anything to get you high, chemically, eventually it burns out. And you want something better, something that'll get you higher, that kind of thing. Or it becomes where you have to have it all the time, even if it's pot or alcohol. It's like you have to have it to get through the day after a while. And you will do anything to get it if you have to have it. I promise, you will do anything.

I mean, you know, robbing, stealing. I mean, I would go in neighborhoods to get drugs where you have to be out of your mind to go in—and I was, literally, out of my mind. I had a gang of guys jump me and take my car, try to run me over with my own car. You know, just things that are all related to drugs. I was in places that I shouldn't been, you know, walking at all hours in the morning to get my drugs. Just putting myself in situations that I would never get into today. And that kind of thing doesn't sound believable when you first start. And that doesn't mean that everybody that has their first drink's gonna be an alcoholic, but it could happen. What people think is that there's an age group or a race group or whatever, but it hits everybody and anybody it wants to, and that's it. There's no restrictions. It's not prejudiced whatsoever. And so you just never know.

You know, I've really learned a lot in the last few months. Maybe it's stuff that other people already know. It's like an inner peace. I go to bed at night and I just thank God that I'm clean and sober. Even if the whole day was just rotten, you know, I always have something. That's what I mean by an inner peace—a happiness where I can appreciate things. I mean, I may have gotten in a car wreck, lost my car, got a ticket, whatever, but I can see that's not such a big deal like it was. I was so wrapped up in the material world and so wrapped up in me, and I had to have this and I had to have that, and then when I didn't get it, I had to get high—then it was like I had something, 'cause I was high.

# CHUCK

**"I just hope that your low point ain't your death; I hope your bottom's not death."**

My dad said the first time I got drunk must've been about when I learned how to walk. It was always when my parents had company over. Even when I was just a little kid, like five or six, I'd always ask, "Dad, can I have a sip of your beer?" And he'd say, "Yeah, just a sip." My dad was an alcoholic. He'd drink a lot. Especially at parties, he'd drink about a six-pack. My mom's not a drinker at all, though. She say, "Stop that." I'd go, "Okay, Mom, I'll stop." And I remember when I was about like fifth grade, I usually got two beers out of the refrigerator and took 'em to my room to drink. I really got off on that. Just by myself. I'd jump around and play. I was always by myself, you know. I had a brother, but he was always—see what it was, I was never good in school. I always got C's and D's and stuff, and my brother was a straight-A student. He's two years younger than I am. I always thought I never was good in anything. Like sports. I never was good in sports. I was the last one to be picked. Always was the last one. That made me mad. In school, I always daydreamed. Just kick back. I used to draw a lot. Not anymore, though. I never draw now. The last time I really drew was when I was in ninth grade. This school I was going to had about three hundred people, and out of three hundred, I got the top prize for my drawings. I think it was eleven—between ten and fifteen drawings I put in, I got 'em all first place.

Chuck, eighteen, came from a middle-class surburban family. He admits battling a lifelong shyness problem, one that made him look constantly for acceptance; his easygoing manner is only a cover-up. He said that his parents were good parents, that they loved him and "did the best they could. They didn't make me get good grades or anything like that in order to love me, like some kids' parents I know, who wouldn't be nice to their kids unless they did good on something."

My parents never caught me sneaking beers. I'd just go in the refrigerator and get 'em out and take 'em to my room. I never felt like I was doing anything wrong. After I finished 'em, I'd just smush the cans, put 'em in my pocket, and throw 'em in the trash can when no one was looking. I used to get away with it. I used to get away with a lot of stuff.

These guys I used to hang around with, you know, these guys were my friends ever since first grade. This one guy, he taught me how to tie my shoes. He was one of the punkers, one of the first punkers. This was about seventh grade. But I wasn't really into it in the seventh grade, I really didn't get—I was in and out, you know. I hung around with a whole lot of punkers. This guy Jeff, he had a shaved head and wore flannel shoes. I had my long hair, and stuff like that. I didn't know what I was in then, you know, I'd just listen to anything. I remember, in seventh grade I used to hang around two crowds: longhairs and punkers. I hung with the people that listened to heavy metal and all that; only it wasn't called heavy metal then, it was called acid rock—all stuff from the sixties. And I didn't even like the music, I just hung around 'cause I wanted to be accepted. Like Led Zeppelin. I don't know, I forced myself to listen to Led Zeppelin. I don't like Led Zeppelin. I really don't, it's not my thing. But, you know, when Jeff would get punk tapes I got off on that, I liked punk. Some of the stuff I sort of forced myself to like, but there's some of it I did like: "Wasted Youth." When I heard that, man, I loved that stuff. This was about 1981. I still have the album. That's how I got over the shyness, was by drinking and just, you know, being with people.

In the ninth grade, I got a haircut, real short, a crew cut, you know, punk style. What happened was, I'd gone to this party, this little punk party. I told my mom I was going to a dance at school and friends were gonna pick me up. My friends weren't old enough to drive, so I told her it was Jeff's brother—but he didn't have a brother. So we went down to the party, and after the party went to this club to see a punk band. I was so scared. All these guys, punks, you know, and I'm sitting there at the bar all by myself; I was just watching the band and everyone's going all crazy like that. And these guys—they looked like they were in high school, about three or four years older—started pickin' on me. I don't remember what they were saying, but they're picking on me and stuff: "Hey you, longhair, get a haircut, you dumbshit hippie. It's 1980, can't you afford a fucking haircut?" I didn't drink there, I was too afraid. I just wanted to make sure I was aware 'cause I was pretty scared. They were serving young kids too.

I didn't go to another gig for about a year—until I was in the end of eighth grade. I think it was during the summer. We went to see this local punk band. I don't remember where, but I got really blitzed. Beer and pills. I got really sick. A lot of people were smoking pot then, but I didn't smoke any pot until tenth grade. I was too afraid to try it. I guess pills didn't bother me, though. I got sort of talked into them. This girl that I sort of fell in love with—she didn't really like me, but I sort of liked her—goes, "Try these." I go, "Okay." Black beauties. And I think some yellow jackets too. Uppers. And Valiums. I remember one incident when I was in ninth grade. I took a lot of Valiums and I ate a lot of food and I was getting really sick, and I puked right in the middle of English class. You know, I never got her, this girl, to like me. If it'd been a friend giving them to me, I probably wouldn't have taken them. But I wanted to impress her—impress her to be like one of the group, to be like her. I saw a picture in the annual just a while ago, and she wasn't that good-looking at all. She didn't grow up to be too good-looking.

Chuck began attending more punk clubs, telling his parents any sort of story he thought they might believe to account for his absences. And while his drug usage and club-hopping together obviously changed his personality, his parents didn't seem to notice. "I think," he said, "they were in denial."

Two of us would like put in for a six-pack—put in a buck and get three beers. You know, it was like our lunch money, so we'd buy the cheapest brew around, you know, have someone buy it for us—hang out in front of the liquor store. We'd have a six-pack on Fridays, Friday night, Friday after school. We'd go down where all the clubs were for just like a couple of hours and drink down there. All of the punkers were there. I wasn't completely a punker then, I was jumping in and out; when I was around the punks I acted like the punks, and then when I would hang around with the longhairs I acted like a longhair. I just threw my image wherever it was going—wherever I was accepted, that's how I acted.

At that time, I was doing just the basics—you know, the pills and everything—and then when I got in ninth grade I sort of died off the pills and I just drank instead. I think I was drinking a six-pack by myself by then. What I'd do is, I'd just like go out and drink, and I used to wait till the buzz was over, until I was really blitzed and could sort of crash. I'd go to a friend's house, brush my teeth, and go home. This one guy, Jeff, was the guy I knew, and I'd go to his house, and his mom didn't come home until like eight or nine. His real punk-rock friends came over. This guy named Ted would come over, and then he'd usually leave me hanging. It was like, when someone else was around, forget Chuck, you know.

The summer after my last year in junior high, ninth

grade, before I went to high school, I drank on just the weekends or with my friend across the street that I knew since I was in about fourth grade. I used to drink with him. Sometimes we'd get into my father's liquor, to make vodka and orange juice. But I really didn't like hard liquor. I always went, "Where's the beer?" I always went and got the beers. Dad always had like a case of beer in there. And over the summer, I sort of got out of punk, you know. 'Cause I grew out my hair again. So I got out of the punk image a little. And I was listening to Van Halen and all that stuff, you know, and I just liked it. Except for when high school started. I was very intimidated by everybody. It was a very jock-oriented school, this all-boys Catholic school, and I wasn't that good in sports. So I just shined them all; I had hair that was down to my neck and I just shaved it the second week of school. I just one day took the bus down home, and I go, "Mom, can I borrow six bucks? I'm gonna get a haircut." I came home with a shaved head. I just told the barber I want a crew cut. And he goes, "Are you sure?" And I go, "Yeah, I mean all off." Like military style, I guess you would say. I was going, "Yeah, now like this, this is better." My dad goes, "Oh, you look like your grandpa, ha-ha," 'cause my gramps has always had a crew cut. He didn't know what was going on in the punk scene, so he didn't get it. It was kind of funny that he thought I looked like gramps. 'Cause when I was in eighth grade, I bought a couple punk records, like Black Flag's first album and Bad Religion's first album. And I was listening to the stuff, and my mom got really angry with me one time 'cause I wasn't doing the chores she asked me to do. And I sort of ran off the mouth, you know, cussing her out. And she slapped me; she came to my room and broke my records, and that's—I remember that. She thought my mouthing off had something to do with listening to that music. I guess she was pretty perceptive.

I was punked. I'd hang by myself, and I didn't really have any friends there. I'd just hang by myself, most of the time. I felt so much different than everyone else anyway, and goin' punk really magnified that. There was this one guy I made friends with, finally—well, tenth grade, I guess. You know, people will talk to you like at lunch time, you talk to 'em and blow them off. Then, middle of tenth grade, I met these guys that I used to know, that I hung around, people I used to meet when I was going down to the clubs when I was in junior high. I started hanging around with them, and so after school they would be in the supermarket parking lot, so I'd go with them. We'd go down to Hollywood and come back, like, ten or eleven o'clock. My parents were suckers. I always told them I'm just at someone's house. I didn't do this on an everyday basis, it was like twice a week. Friday nights and Tuesday nights. So anyway, we'd go to this club. Tuesday night was dollar night. We used to hang around and drink and stuff. They didn't give a shit how old you were, if you were under drinking age; a couple years later they were closed down for violence and serving alcohol to minors. So I'd just hang around with these guys. I'd meet, like, two of them in a car, and I'd take it down to where there was like a bunch of us, and most of it was girls—about like eleven girls and about, like, five or six of us guys. Most of 'em were like brothers and sisters that knew each other; like, three of 'em were brothers, one had like two sisters, and the other had three sisters. Just hanging around with a bunch of little punkers drinking beer at this place.

I was sort of like the mascot, you know. I was younger, and there were some that were my age, but I was the smallest of 'em, you know, and they used to pick on me a lot and stuff like that. They're going, "Oh, we gotta make you a man," and they used to beat me up and stuff like that. Sometimes they'd start off kidding around and they'd start punching me and stuff like that. I don't know why I let them do it; I kept going 'cause it's the only friends—and I sort of felt like I deserved it, 'cause I felt like I was a wimp and shit like that. All my life I always felt like I was less than everyone else, 'cause I never thought I was that good. I always compared myself to other people: "Well, I'm not as good as them so I won't even try." One of the things I'm going through right now is trying to figure all this shit out.

I remember when I was probably in first grade, and second grade, we'd have spelling tests. I gotta spell "could" and "would," and I remember I'd be taking a bath and my dad would come in with his little miniature chalk board: "This is how you spell these things, right?" And I would try to, and it would take me a half an hour just to get all these words right, you know. And I always quit. I'd go, "No, I can't do this, forget it, so and so will get the A. I'm not gonna get the A." And from being a little kid, it just picked up, you know, and I was always saying, "Oh, I'm not that"—especially with sports. I'd go, "I'm not good in sports, so you know I suck, so why you wanna pick me?" I sort of made myself suck, I guess. I'd probably've been good. I guess people just sort of picked up the vibes after a while. I mean, you didn't have to be a genius. I believed it and they believed it, and you know how kids get. You know, elementary school. "I'm not good in this." "Yeah, you're right, you're not."

With my punk friends, I'd invited it big-time. 'Cause I wasn't that strong. I was a skinny little kid. They'd pick on me: "Well, that'll make you tough." I remember a couple situations I would fight back and they would push me on the ground and kick me. They didn't like it when I fought back, but I thought that was the purpose of the thing. That's what I thought at the beginning. After that, I just let them pick on me. They did that twice, and I just let them pick on me. I never told anybody, and I never told them to leave me alone, and I just hung with them 'cause they were my only friends.

Not surprisingly, Chuck's association with his "friends" led to a lot of drinking—and other drugs.

I could drink a twelve-pack, no problem. I'd be pretty blitzed—a little sloppy, maybe—but I could hold my own. Sometimes I'd get sick, unless I didn't eat that much, or if I mixed something with it, some pills and stuff, mix it like that, I could handle it. During the summer a situation happened with one of the guys that used to beat me up, this guy Jay. Him and me was kicking back for a day, until we were gonna go to the cafe that night, and we're just kicking around and stuff, and he goes, "What are we gonna do, wanna get some beer? I'm gonna get some fry." That's acid; they call it fry 'cause it fries your brain. Well, I didn't want to do it ever, 'cause it was a little scary for me, but this time I wanted to do it. I guess I'd started smoking pot a little while before that. You know, they were like, "Here, it's a joint, smoke it," so I had to do it. I kind of liked it, though, so I guess in a way that made me want to do the acid.

And so we go and fry. We go to this house, where he lives, and we're frying. He was black, and he lived in this area where there were a lot of Mexicans, and it was funny, 'cause they used to pick on him 'cause he was black, I guess. I saw that, when we were walkin' there, and I go, "Whoa." And we go into his place, and we're just tripping. I was tripping hard. I was getting a little scared and stuff. Then all of a sudden out of this, like, credenza he pulls out a gun, and he's fucking around with the gun, and he points at me and it goes click. And I was saying, "Let me see that," and he goes, "No. Okay, you wanna see it?" And he goes click, right at me. It was like one of the police ones, revolvers, you know? Then he puts it to his head and blows his head out. He was trippin' out and he just went "Bam!" You know, the gun probably didn't have all the bullets, 'cause it would have blown my head off. Then he went to his head, I guess assuming it was empty, and went boom. And it blew. And all I saw was red. Red flew on my face. Then I just started trippin' out and I ran all the way home. I just lived about like two miles from his house. I ran all the way home. I just went, got home, and I just—I was just trippin'. My parents go, "What's wrong?" And I go, "Nothing, nothing." I got up to my room and I started to cry and just cried and cried; I don't know for how long. I didn't call the police. I just took a shower and I just went to sleep. And I never went back.

What happened is that, you know, the coroner comes and he said it was suicide. So about two days later, I took a bus down, it was during the summer, and told everybody what happened. They go, "We already know." And they blamed it on me. They go, "Yeah, you killed him, you killed him." And they all beat me up. They beat me up pretty good. I had a bloody nose, got bruises all over; I didn't break anything, though, but I had a black eye. They said I pulled the trigger. When I got home, I told my parents I got in a fight, that somebody tried to take my money, that I'd gotten mugged.

After that I really didn't hang around anybody until after twelfth grade. For about two years I was basically by myself. Through the eleventh and twelfth grades, all I did, I smoked pot and drank beer. I smoked a lot. At the end of the twelfth grade my grades started falling. I mean, in the eleventh grade my grades were shit, but I wanted to graduate, so I stopped smoking pot and kept drinking beer; I don't know if that helped any, but I graduated, you know, and I was still into punk. My parents never knew I was smoking pot, but in the twelfth grade they finally figured out I was drinking. They didn't care. They didn't give a shit. They'd say, "Well, don't drink and drive," and I'd go, "Okay, Mom." By that time, the end of the twelfth grade, I could drink a case of beer by myself. I could drink a lot. Two beers was like water. I was also smoking pot every day. I'd been getting high every day for about two years. I worked at a job in a pizza joint, making pizzas and shit like that. I spent all the money I made on either pot or beer; or the only other I spent was on records or going to gigs. I went to gigs by myself and stuff like that.

In the twelfth grade, Chuck took LSD several times. He did it, he said, because he got it for free from another boy who tried to buy friendships with drugs. "Everybody picked on this guy. He was like the big school loser. He would give me drugs just to have an excuse to hang around me."

My last part of the last half of the twelfth grade, I was drinking about half the days of the week—maybe three to four days of the week I'd be drinking. During school, after school, before school. It didn't matter. My attitude about life was just shit. I didn't care about anything. I used to tell my dad to go fuck off and go and kill himself 'cause he was a loser. I just didn't want his, you know, his love and shit, so I'd just say anything to hurt him. I used to call him a loser a lot. I guess that was a projection; I felt like a loser. I told my mom that she was a whore. I got that from some guy, some pervert who was calling our house and wanted my mom—some fucking breather or something like that. Every time anyone else answered the phone he'd hang up, and every time my mom answered, he'd say all these perverted things, and I called her a whore 'cause of that.

I hated both of them. I hated my brother, hated everybody. I hated myself. I wouldn't even have kept going to school, but they said I would be kicked out of the house if I didn't graduate. I didn't want to go out 'cause I didn't wanna leave the house—you know, free food, free ride. I couldn't get that by myself working at a pizza joint, and anyway most of the money I made I bought beer with. I mean, my paycheck every two weeks lasted four days.

I met this other guy, Joe, who I knew since when I was in first, second, third grade, in this thing called Indian Guides. I met him at this house that José told me about called Mom's House. We used to party there about once every other week. It was this lady's house, she was a coke fiend. I only did coke about three times there, but mostly I just stayed with the acid, beer, and pot. I met this guy over there, Paul. He was into punk, I was into punk, he had no friends, I had no friends, so we made the perfect pair. We drank a lot of beer together, got into a lot of trouble together. We used to get arrested. The first time was in twelfth grade. It was for vandalism, but they dropped charges 'cause they didn't have evidence. What we did was, we used spray paint all over this gas station just for the fuck of it. It was just to prove our punk-rockedness. We sprayed "anarchy" and the names of all our favorite bands on there and stuff like that, and then we stopped and we threw the cans away and sat there and drank more beers. And the cops rolled up, and they said we did it. We said it was already there. They said, "The paint's wet." We said, "It could be anybody around here." So they threw that out, 'cause they didn't have no evidence, 'cause they didn't see it.

The next time I got arrested was waiting for José to get off work. We were broke, and it was the day he was getting paid. He said he'd buy us beer. He went, "I'll buy you a couple of cases." He was celebrating for some reason I don't remember. And he bought two cases of beer, and we drank it, but Paul goes, "That ain't gonna last." So José goes, "Okay, four cases of beer, or how about six?" We go, "Okay." So we drank six cases between us three. We had a twelve-pack of Olde English 800, and we drank all those up and we were just kicking back listening to music in my car, and all of a sudden I hear this guy say, "Put your hands on the car." And I turn around and say, "What did you just say, you fucking asshole?" And I'm assuming—I thought it was José, right? And I turned around, and this cop pulls out his billy club and says, "You say one more word I'm gonna smash you." So he cuffed us and took us down to the station. We were just waiting; we're listening to music, kicking back. We were thrown in the dry tank, and they said they were gonna press charges and all this stuff. We were causing a lot of trouble inside, too. What we'd do, we'd hang off the bars and bang against the door; hang off the top of these, like these grate things, these chain-link fences that they had on the ceiling, and swing back and forth, banging against things. We caused a lot of trouble and stuff. I wasn't scared 'cause I was drunk. I was never scared when I was drunk. When I didn't have any beer in my system, I was scared. Then they told us we each had a phone call to make—this was about four hours later, and I really wanted out of there bad. But I couldn't call my parents, so Paul says he'll go make a call. What he did, he called long distance to Nebraska. I mean, he didn't know anybody there or anything, he just happened to know the area code for Nebraska. So I had to call my mom and dad. "Ah, Dad, I'm gonna be home late." "Why?" "Because I'm in jail." About six hours later he comes and he bails me out. And ever since then, they sort of, like, just gave up on me.

Every time I'd get in arguments, especially like arguing with my mom, I'd take off. They'd take my car keys away and stuff like this when I was in the summer before college. My dad used to follow me. He goes, "Get here in back of the car, get in the back of the car." I go, "Fuck you, get away from me." So I ended up walking out. I guess if I'd been them, dealing with me, I'd have kicked the shit out of me. If I had a kid that was like me, I'd shoot him, I would. Hang him from the nearest tree. They were very lenient. Too lenient. I mean, they were very kick-back.

About the middle of my first semester of junior college, I'd start drinking as soon as I'd wake up. I was drinking beer. This one morning, I remember waking up and I was shaking—going through withdrawals real bad. Then I stopped shaking and started hallucinating, and I said, "Oh, I want some beer." So I went down to the liquor store asked some guy to buy me beer. Ever since then, I always had beer in my room. See, my parents by then already said no more beer in the house, so I drank in the backyard, and that didn't help much. I started drinking every—I always had a beer; I'd drink like a couple beers in the morning, even brush my teeth with beer, even did the corn flakes with beer. I always had a beer. I don't know where I got it. Most of the time we stole it—me and Paul stole from the liquor stores. That's how we got most of our beer—by stealing it. I had this cooler, and I'd throw ice in it and put beers in it. We always had, like, four different brands of beers in there, 'cause you can't select what you steal. One time, I remember, we stole a case of near-beer and just threw it away. We were pissed. We brought it back to the place and threw it in the guy's face. "We didn't want this beer." We stole it and took it back. That was pretty demented. We took it back to him and we stole another one.

I'd always go over to Paul's house. His parents didn't give a shit. They didn't care. We started just throwing the empties in his room, so he's got a carpet of empties in his room, right? So his dad got pissed: "You can't drink inside the house, drink outside the house." So we drank outside. His dad never really punished him. Like, when were in Indian Guides, he'd bounce on couches at people's houses where we had our meetings and his dad would just kinda, like, try to reason with him—not like my mom, who'd go bam. My mom and dad really stopped punishing me, like spanking me or hitting me, when I started in like eighth grade. Probably, if they'd've beat the shit out of me a few more times I'd probably have been a nice little boy.

**Everywhere he went, Chuck drank. He was never without beer.**

I knew I had a problem. I was sick of drinking all the time. I was getting tired of it. I always had a beer, and when I didn't have that beer, I'd go berserk—and I didn't like the feeling. By this time we'd picked up a couple of friends: this guy named Howard, and this little midget guy; we called him Fidget, the chicken hawk. He had a haircut like a chicken hawk. Howard knew this girl he'd been flirting with might get us free food at this bowling alley, right? So we go over there, expecting to get some free food, and all we see is these bunch of bikers and we're going, "Oh, shit." And they started, "Oh you stupid punk rockers, you bunch of lame old pieces of shit," and they're all carrying on like that, and we're all, "Oh, fuck you, get away from us, we're just coming here to get something to eat, now leave us alone." And they're pushing us around and stuff, right? And they threw us out of the bowling alley. So we go, "Fuck you," and stuff like that. This little guy, Fidget, he started the whole thing. He was a wrestler, he weighed about 210, even though he only came up to about my chest. He was all muscle, no fat, but he looked funny 'cause he walked funny. Well, he started it. He jumped on one guy and started pounding on his face, right? We're going, "Oh, shit."

So we pulled him off and got in our car, and the bikers start throwing beer bottles at my car, at my Volkswagen bug. They were throwing beer bottles, beer cans, and probably Pepsi cans and Pepsi bottles and whatever, throwing shit at my car, right? So I got really pissed and started driving my car toward the bikes—all these Harleys. And I hit 'em, and they all, like dominoes, seven bikes went, like that. This guy came over and tried to wreck my car, so I backed up and hit him, 'cause I'd just replaced the fender. He fell on the ground and bumped his head; he was out cold on the cement. So we took off and one guy on his motorcycle came following us, and then I slammed on the brakes. He hit the bumper and fell off, so then we go off, right? What did we do? We stole more beer, went out drinking somewhere where I guess all these devil-worshipers go, and we're drinking, and we go, "Fuck this, let's get a Molotov cocktail and bomb them bikes." We didn't think what we did was good enough.

We went back home—almost drove off a cliff going through a canyon, and went to Howard's house. We took an old Kahlua bottle his grandma had, collected all our pennies together to buy some gasoline, and put a diaper in the neck of the bottle. Then we went back and what we did, we spray-painted "Punk's Not Dead" on the walls right above the motorcyles while the bikers were inside, and Fidget lit the diaper and threw the Molotov at all the bikes. I can't believe how demented that was. They all blew up or caught on fire or whatever. We just took off and went home.

If I wasn't drinking, I wouldn't have done stuff like that, no way. That was so demented, but I didn't know what I was doing. I was trying to prove myself, and it's sort of like, you know, a mob-like little incident. It was a mobby kind of thing you do—anything that the mob does, just be one of the guys.

**After the incident in the bowling alley parking lot, Chuck decided he needed help to stop drinking.**

I was driving home after I dumped everybody off and I was drinking beer and I just looked at this beer and I said, "Fuck this shit, I can't handle this. Why am I doing this? I never did this before." I don't know, it's just like I just took a look at my life and went, "What the hell am I doing?" I went home and told my mom to help me. She said, "We've been looking at this place, this rehab place, for a few months. Why don't you take a look at it?" I guess they'd been waiting for me to come to them, 'cause I was eighteen at the time and they couldn't threw me in a detox hospital then. I guess they could've kicked me out of the house, which would probably have woke me up.

When I first went, I said, "Okay, I'll just give this a try," you know? I stayed sober for about like a month or two months. It felt good, but it was scary. But I was bored. I didn't know how to have fun without drinking. So I just popped over to Paul's house and I'm going, "Hey, what's going on?" And I drank. We just kept it at his house. We had fun, fun and stuff. But when I got home like in the morning, I went through withdrawals again—sweaty, really like cold sweat, I guess, and shaking. The one thing I thought was fun about my withdrawals was holding a glass of water. I don't know, I didn't think that was weird, I thought it was pretty neat, 'cause I looked at it and I just freaked out. I had no control. Then I would hallucinate, feeling like things were crawling up my legs and stuff. I remember once in my drafting class, another time that I slipped, everything suddenly got real little, and all of a sudden I felt things crawling up my leg. I was brushing 'em off, and I was just having this fit, and I just took off class and I went home. I left my equipment and stuff on the table.

Chuck "slipped" several other times, taking heroin and smoking crack along with beer drinking, before staying sober; it's now been a year. He has developed an almost messianic zeal for passing along the lessons he learned the hard way. Yet he's realistic enough to know that other kids contemplating drug use rarely listen to others, even those who've used.

Drugs, drugs, they don't do anything good to you—just get you sick, that's all. But if you really wanna use drugs, I just hope that your low point ain't your death; I hope your bottom's not death.

# SANDI

**"I thought I was like everybody else. I thought I was just an ordinary teenage kid. I didn't know there was something wrong, and I didn't know it was drugs and alcohol. I had no idea that drugs and happiness were incompatible."**

I started drinking when I was about eleven years old at Temple. They call kids up for children's prayers, and they give out little, like, shot glasses of wine. I can look back now and I see how I used to wait to be the last person, so that there's extras on the tray. I started drinking just like shot glasses of wine at Temple and then when I started going to Bar and Bat Mitzvahs, we used to like joke around and kid around: "Let's sneak the wine off the parents' table." We used to do it all together. I used to get really out of hand, and I'd go home totally obliterated. My parents didn't know—at least now they say they didn't know—but I don't see how they couldn't notice. You know, a twelve- or thirteen-year-old girl coming home totally drunk.

Sandi, nineteen, is the adopted daughter of an upper-middle-class family. She has a brother who is four years older than she. Both of them, she admitted, were spoiled.

I never hung around the girls at my temple, 'cause they all thought I was a snob. I didn't feel real comfortable, 'cause the Temple wasn't, like, a wealthy Temple, and a lot of the girls' mothers would like make them dresses for Bar and Bat Mitzvahs, and I always could go buy something. I don't think I was a snob, I don't think I acted like a snob until the girls were telling me I was a snob and that I was a bitch so much that I started acting that way. What happened was, I started drawing more towards the guys. And a lot of the guys were like two years older than me, and so then I started going out on dates with them. I guess I was about thirteen or fourteen, and they were sixteen, so they could drive. They would come pick me up, and we would go and get drunk.

Through my whole schooling years, I never felt like I belonged anywhere. And when I got drunk I felt like I was okay with myself, and I could be whoever I wanted to be and I could act any way I wanted to, and that I was acceptable. If I wasn't drunk or high, I think I felt like I wasn't good enough, or I wasn't pretty enough, or I didn't wear the right clothes, or I didn't hang around the right crowd of people. I always was looking at that, like, popular crowd to fit into. There's always that one group, this one clique, that you see that always seems to be having this totally wild time and having fun, and I was always looking at that wanting to be there. And I wasn't there. I just kinda hung out on the sidelines, with a bunch of other friends. This was at school that I mainly felt that way. At Temple, I started feeling like I was better than them. So it was weird, 'cause at school I felt inferior, and at Temple I felt superior, which was how they made me feel. At Temple I got a reputation like I was a sleaze—you know, I wasn't a nice girl, 'cause I was always with the guys. I was hanging all over the guys. I felt I got a lot of attention from them, and I felt like I was more mature than the girls at the temple. The guys would say, "Oh, you're more mature than them, you're not sitting around gossiping about people and stuff like that." So I really liked that attention that I got from them, and I really fed into it. I learned how to manipulate guys at a really young age.

Sandi's feelings of worthlessness and inferiority were exacerbated at home, where she believed she was supposed to live up to the high standards her brother had set.

I was a competitive swimmer since I was like six, and my brother was a competitive swimmer. There was, like, a pressure between me and my brother. I always felt like I had to live up to my brother's expectations; whatever he was doing, I was supposed to follow in his steps, 'cause he was like a straight-A student. And I wasn't very good with school. I didn't get very good grades. I had a learning disability, mostly in math; I just couldn't comprehend what was being taught. And we didn't find this out till years later, when I was already too old to start learning how to learn easier. What happened was, I was like failing in math all the time, and I was having tutors and nothing was working, so my parents had me go to a place where they give out tests to see what your abilities are in certain classes. And math was like way down. I was like in tenth grade or something, doing fifth-grade math. English I excelled in, but math I didn't. My dad would say things like—I would be so proud to come home with, like, a ninety-eight percent on a spelling test or something—"Well, if you studied an hour longer, you could've got a hundred percent." So it made me feel like I was never good enough for Daddy.

At fourteen, Sandi started smoking pot with some of the kids at school.

I was smoking it whenever someone had it, basically. Not, like, mass quantities, but I'd smoke it on the weekends. Around that time I started slipping away from Temple; I stopped going there altogether. I'd had my Bat Mitzvah the year before, and then, like, right after that I didn't go to Temple anymore, and I didn't hang around the people at Temple. So all those friends were gone, and then I started hanging out with the kids at school. And I started hanging out with the crowd that I wanted to hang out with—the one I thought was totally cool. What happened was, one of my friends started hanging around this girl and we all got high together. So that made us friends, too. Then it was like, okay, we're in. Well, we weren't totally in, and I still didn't feel like I was part of the crowd, you know. I don't know. I was kinda in, and kinda not, and I felt so bad 'cause it wasn't working out like it was supposed to. And around that time I slit my wrist at school, 'cause I just felt like dying. I did it at school with this metal thing off a pen cap. I don't really remember what I was thinking at the time. I think I just started cutting myself sort of, just like scratching hard, and then while I was doing it, I started getting deeper and deeper. I was in class. I was just kinda rubbing it on my skin, and then I just started gouging in really deep. It wasn't like totally deep or anything, but there was a pretty big slash on my wrist. I didn't hit a vein or anything, so it didn't spurt blood. It was basically, I think, self-destruction. When the blood started coming out, I had to go get paper towels and stuff, so I just left the room. Our school was, like, really lenient. It was this weird private school. If we didn't want to do our work we didn't have to. You pay the money, and if you don't want to do the work you don't have to do it. I put a bunch of Band-Aids on it, and when my parents asked me what happened, I said I fell on a tree branch on the way to the park.

I always felt like I never belonged anywhere. Actually, I'm not really sure still if I was trying to kill myself or if I just wanted attention. I think I might have just wanted attention. I was very . . . I really needed a lot, a lot of attention. And I wasn't getting it. Actually, I don't know if I wasn't getting attention, I just wasn't getting the kind of attention I wanted. I wanted attention from guys. I wanted more attention than I was getting. I became totally obsessed. It's like I always needed that attention from men, and that recognition, and if I didn't get it, then I would do something to get it. If I had to hurt myself, I would hurt myself. I mostly hung around guys, and they would find out I was hurt, and they would come talk to me and go, "Oh, what did you do, why did you do this, don't you know we care about you?" And so I'd be like that. The only people I told about it were these guys Matt and Buster. They were real sweet.

I'd started sleeping around at the Temple with the guys there when I was thirteen. I was hanging all over these guys, and I think I felt like I had to do it. 'Cause it seemed like they were thinking, "She wouldn't do that," so it was kinda like in my head, "Well, I'm gonna show them that I would." So I did it with one guy, and he went and told all his other friends, so then it was like they all started coming on to me real heavy. Like, I'd go out with someone else, and they'd come on to me really heavy, and I would just go with them too. I liked it. I was high all the time when I did it. It was kinda like, get drunk and get it on. I never did it straight.

A couple weeks after the thing with my wrist I ate a bunch of aspirin. First I went to my friend, I think it was Molly. I kept going, "Can I have some aspirin, you know? I have a headache." And so she gave me some. I said, "Can I have two more?" So she gave me some more. Then I went to Matt and Buster and said, "Do you have any aspirin?" And Beth was standing there. She said, "Well, she already took four." And Buster said, "You can't take any more, you know, you're gonna get sick." And I said, "No I'm not." So they were kind of like following me around school, but I ended up finding a few more aspirins and I took them. I ended up getting really sick, and they called me in the office 'cause someone said I was trying to commit suicide, and I said, "No, no, no, I wasn't, you know, I just feel really sick today." So they let me go, and then Matt and Buster took me in the bathroom, and one of them stuck his fingers down my throat and made me throw it all up. And they just, you know, they're like, "I can't believe you're doing this. What are you doing to yourself?" Every day at school, they'd come up to me and ask me how I was doing, so I really got attention from those two guys. They were always asking how I was. They were always giving me hugs. They were always giving me physical attention—hugging, kissing, and stuff, at school, in front of people. That made me feel like someone really cared. I don't know what I thought. It's hard for me now to look back and see what I was really thinking or what I was really trying to do with the aspirin and the pen cap. At the time I thought I was trying to kill myself, but I think, looking back, a lot of it had to do with wanting attention from people.

Since she's been sober, Sandi said, she's been trying to evaluate some of the motives for her past actions. One pattern she noticed was an inability to get close to people emotionally. She attributes that to her adoption. "I feel," she said, "like people are always going to leave me."

A weird thing I found out was that some people I had been drawn to were adopted, and I didn't even know it at the time; I wouldn't know they were adopted until after we talked. When I was in grade school, it was, like, people would start talking about adopted kids for some reason or another, and I would say, "Oh, I was adopted," 'cause I thought it was special to be adopted. You know, I thought I was special. I was picked, and I was chosen, and then everyone started calling me a bad girl, you know, "Mommy gave you away." So that started going in my head. I thought I was a bad girl from a very young age.

I wasn't really close to anyone really in my family. I just kind of came home from school and went into my room. I didn't even talk that much, I don't think, to my parents. I wished they would've talked to me more. They used to ask me like, "Oh, did you do your homework, how was school, how was swimming?" And I'd be like, "Fine, fine, fine." And I would just like disappear in my room until it was time for dinner. I'd come down, eat dinner, and then go back into my room. So I didn't really spend time with the family, and I just kinda like isolated in my room. And I didn't even feel like it was my room. I had this big huge walk-in closet, and the back part of it was all clear, so I made like a little clubhouse thing in there. I brought my radio in there and my telephone and hung up posters in there and pillows and stuff, and that was where I felt okay. Which is sad, to think that your daughter's living in a closet. They never thought anything weird about it, I guess. They just thought I wanted a little clubhouse or something. I wish they would've asked me why I was in there. I guess I could've gone up to them too, but I still wish they would've asked me. I don't think that's a normal thing, for kids to be in their closets a lot. I mean, maybe if you find a kid in your closet once in a while playing with their toys or something. But I just used to sit in there and stare at the walls.

At fifteen, Sandi started sneaking liquor occasionally from her parents' cabinet.

I wasn't drinking that much and I was only getting high if it was at school. We used to get high behind the buildings. But when I did drink I was getting heavily loaded. Weekends was when I'd get obliterated. That lasted about the whole year, the whole ninth grade, and by the end of the year I was like getting high not every day, but sporadically through the week. And then summer came and I was smoking it almost all the time. My parents didn't find out—at least, they say they didn't know. I guess it might've been their denial or their unawareness of drugs. They didn't use anything themselves. My dad had a gin and tonic once in a while, and my mother doesn't drink anything.

When I changed from junior high school to high school at the end of that summer, I just felt lost altogether. It was a big public school, and I was like, "Oh, my God." There were people I knew, I just felt like I didn't belong. It was so big. I saw people I hadn't seen since fourth grade and stuff, but I didn't really know them. I saw a lot of people that went to my elementary school when I was in fourth grade, and I reunited with them. I started getting high with them and then I started meeting other people. I guess all my friendships, or relationships or whatever, were based on drugs. You know, here it was again, I want to be in THE popular crowd at high school, and the only thing that looked appealing was to be a cheerleader. So I decided I was gonna become a cheerleader. And I wasn't doing it to go be spirited about the school and stuff. I thought the uniforms were really cute, and I liked the crowd of people that I saw. And you know, the cheerleaders seemed to be popular; they seemed to be getting all the attention from everybody, and they seemed to be getting special privileges. You know, all the football players kind of came on to them, and I didn't care about the football players, really; it's just that they were the popular guys. I didn't even know anything about sports, barely, except swimming. And I was also on the swim team. It's not easy swimming when you're loaded pretty much all the time, but I managed. We have a pool at home, so I had a lot of practice. Pretty soon, though, I started not swimming. I started telling my mom I was going to work out, and I would skip and go out with my friends, and I'd like wet my bathing suit and stash it in my bag and damp my towel, and, "My eyes are red because I was swimming, Mom. The chlorine, you know, it's like killing my eyes."

So I was getting high all the time, every day in tenth grade. And I was cheerleading. I made it on the cheerleading squad, and I was seeing there were all these new people, and it was like, "God, this is great." And I got attention. So I felt really good, and after a while it was like I felt really good that I belonged where I did, and I seemed to get along with everybody. And what I noticed was that everybody was like really stuck-up; there was like a lot of back-stabbing going on. The people were like, "If you don't hang out with this group of friends, you're like not cool for us, you know, and like this crowd doesn't go out with the people over here with long hair, and the longhairs don't go out with the punks, and the punks aren't going out with the cheerleaders," and I never felt like I had anything against any of the other crowds of people, but I wasn't supposed to like these people or those people. And I hated it.

That was the year my brother went to college, so I started going to his fraternity parties. I was having a blast. It was like, "God, here I am, tenth grade, going to these college parties. I'm cool." I always looked older than my age, and I never wanted to be my age, so I always acted older, and so in tenth grade I was going to fraternity parties. Me and my friend would stay in the fraternity house with the guys. I mean, we were walking into fraternity houses and looking at the names on the directory, and we'd go, "Oh, is David here?" That's how we would meet people. We'd walk into a fraternity house, and we'd be like, "Well, who's gonna turn away two pretty girls that come strolling on in?" And they'd go, "Oh, he's upstairs in room whatever, you know, down and to the left." So we'd start meeting people that way. We'd just walk into fraternity houses. When we'd go to my brother's parties, I think he thought it was cute, 'cause his little sister was drunk. He was loaded too. I'd started smoking weed with him a couple years before, so I got big brother loaded on weed for his first time.

It was a babysitter that was staying at my house that turned me on the first time. My parents were away—they were always going away. Like, once a year they'd go away for three and a half weeks or four weeks for my dad's business. It's like a worldwide convention that they have and all the offices come. And so they'd leave me, they'd leave us with different sitters. This one year this young couple that had stayed with my cousins stayed with us. My cousins seemed to really enjoy them staying with them, so my parents had them stay with me. And I was going, "Hmm, there's a reason they enjoy them, 'cause Nancy doesn't get along with too many people." So they stayed with me and they gave me this weed to smoke and I was like all nervous and stuff, but I was really excited 'cause I knew the kids at school were doing it, and I didn't have to do it in front of the kids at school, so by the time I did it with the kids at school I already knew how. I was like, I was cool, and I felt right. I was going to high school and going to the college parties, and I thought I was better than my high school friends, 'cause I was going to fraternity parties. It's like, "I'm gonna bring my fraternity guy with me."

See, it was like I lost track along the way from when I started sleeping around at Temple—who was a boyfriend and who was a friend. So I'd have my boyfriend here, and I would sleep with him and have a relationship with him, but yet my friend over here, I was sleepin' with him too. I lost track of what things you were supposed to do with your boyfriends and what things you're not supposed to do. So it was like my boyfriends were the same as my friends. I didn't know what was going on. I had no values, and I didn't care; as long as I got high and I got drunk I didn't care what I did, and that's how it was in tenth grade.

Ever since I was twelve years old I wanted to be a call girl. It's like, where did I get that in my head? I have no idea how I knew about call girls. Maybe TV or something, maybe in a TV movie. I mean that's the only place I can think I saw it. I have no idea, but all I know is, I wanted to be a call girl because I thought that was glamorous, and you get gifts, and you get money, and you have men at your feet, and it was like I knew that at twelve. I started developing that then myself. I wasn't getting gifts and stuff, but it was like, if I got my drugs and I got high, then I'd do what you want me to do. The second semester I was a cheerleader, I sprained my ankle, but I didn't really care anyhow 'cause I just liked flashing the skirt around. Ever since I got that thought in my head at twelve, it seems like the rest of my years of dressing was more to appeal to men than it was what I liked myself. It was kinda like, "Well, I'll wear the shortest skirt I can find, and if they like it, you know, that's cool. If they don't like it, I'll find something else." So I dressed to please men. There was never a time when a boy or man came on to me that I said no to him. Never.

By the eleventh grade, Sandi was getting high every day and staying high all day long. "I could care less if I went to class," she said. "Mostly I ditched school." Her parents still were unaware of her drug use. "Their denial was so heavy."

I stole money from my dad whenever I didn't have money to buy booze or drugs. I'd just take a twenty out of his wallet and leave. It's kinda like he was unconscious, 'cause there was one time I took two hundred dollars out of his wallet and he didn't know. And to this day I don't think he even knows. But I never really had to worry about money for anything besides drugs. They, my parents, gave me all the money I needed for clothes and meals and movies and stuff like that. I never had to work. I was totally irresponsible. My parents took care of everything. It was like, if I got in trouble at school, Mom would come in and patch it all up. She started working at my school as a volunteer in tenth grade, and my grades were bad, and she'd go and talk to the teachers: "Can you please just give her a D?" And they'd raise my grade. I kinda got the message that anything goes, that I'll always get bailed out.

I'd already starting snorting coke, 'cause I did it at my brother's frat house. He was totally against it, and he said if he ever found out anyone was giving me cocaine, he would kill them. Me and my friend were like running to these two guys at the frat house who kept feeding us cocaine; we were snorting it all and running around like spastics. And I really didn't like what cocaine did to me. I liked more like feeling down and low—downers and stuff. But after that first weekend doing coke, when I came home I was like, "Oh, my God, give me more, I want some more cocaine." I was totally obsessed on this new drug, 'cause it was new. That was my addictive personality right there. I didn't even like it and I was doing it, and I was almost in tears with my best friend. I was like, "I need some cocaine and I need it now."

**That fall, when her parents went away for three weeks to attend her father's annual convention, they left her in the care of a twenty-one-year-old girl.**

Perfect. Yay. You know, I was thrilled to death, 'cause this girl wasn't gonna tell me what to do. She wasn't old enough to tell me what to do. She's twenty-one, perfect to go buy alcohol. It works out perfectly, and she did, 'cause she didn't know how to control me. She had no idea how to control me. I did what I wanted to, and she'd tell me to be home at this time, but I'd come home whenever I wanted to. She left a lot of the times and stayed with her friends. I don't think she liked the scene that was going on. I handed out my house key to a couple of my friends, and I said, you know, "If I'm not home, just come on in and make yourself at home." So it's like my house, you know, cool, everyone come on over and party. And that's what it was, it was like a three-week party. I didn't go to school. I mean, I would go off and on; I'd go to certain classes, the ones I'd get busted in, you know, and other classes; I'd just come in, sign in, and sneak out; and, you know, I'd forge notes and stuff.

I started seeing this guy Tim while all this was going on, and my friends did not like him. He was just some guy that hung around with some of the other crowds. He was a grade older than me, and he wasn't part of the group, he wasn't part of the scene with the cheerleaders and football players and the snobs and the cool guys in their nice cars. He was nice-looking and he didn't give a hot shit about what he wore or the groups he fit in with or stuff like that. So I thought he was really cool. What I didn't know was he had just come out of a drug and alcohol hospital, so he'd just been treated for that, and he had three months clean. Well, here I am, partying my ass off every single day, and we're like really partying in the house. He was a really neat guy when I first met him. He was three months sober and he started hanging around with me and got loaded. He started getting loaded with us again. I mean, I just had parties all the time and had people coming over all the time. We were doing all sorts of drugs. Everything just about you can think of.

When I started seeing Tim, my friends didn't like him at all 'cause once he started partying again he got like really violent—he had a really bad temper. If he didn't get his way, that was it, you know, you just better watch out. But I still liked him. I thought he was cool. You know, "This guy's gonna take care of me, let me tell you, this guy is the one." So I started like, "Well, shine you guys, you know, fuck all of you. If you don't like who I'm seeing, you guys aren't friends to even hang around. You don't have to be with him when we go out, he can go out with his friends." But they didn't like the whole idea. And my friends also started telling me how I was gonna be one of those kids that drop out of the graduating class, you know, and they were watching me fall. I was using more than they were. So I was a drug addict, and I was getting bad in their eyes. Alcohol, pot, cocaine, speed, Valiums. I started doing speed right after cocaine. Whatever was in front of me I would do. And I wouldn't even ask questions. The Valiums I took from my dad. Just one every now and then. Mostly I was smoking weed every single day, and then if cocaine or speed or anything else was around, I would take it. I never did acid or hallucinogenics.

**During the eleventh grade, Sandi started running away from home regularly.**

I was still seeing Tim, and he became very abusive physically and mentally to me. But I guess I didn't care.

He was a guy, and he said he loved me, and I thought I loved him and I could fix him, and it was worse being at home. So when I ran away I'd run to his house. He lived with his parents, but his parents hated my parents. His parents thought my parents were the worst. They thought that my parents didn't know how to control me, that I wasn't a bad kid, that it didn't matter if I used drugs, that it was their fault. And my parents hated Tim. For some reason they hated him from the first moment they saw him. And his parents hated my parents because my parents didn't like him. They didn't know, obviously, that I was using drugs, and they obviously didn't know he was using again. I guess they thought they cleaned up everyone's act. But my parents knew that Tim had been in a drug rehabilitation hospital because I told them. But I told them that he was clean now, though, that that was in the past and can't you let that go? I said, "I can't believe you're putting these things on this poor guy, he's clean now, don't you understand that? He's changing his life." But they hated him, and I believed I loved this guy. So it was like my parents didn't like him, so they didn't want me going out with him, so I went out with him anyhow, and I'd get grounded. So I didn't want to be grounded, so I'd leave anyhow. If they didn't let me go to a party I wanted to go to, I'd go to the party anyhow. I'd leave notes saying, "I went to this party, I'll be home later." And I'd never come home. I'd like come home two days later, because once I was out, it's like once I was high, once I was just so fucked up—I was taking everything I could get my hands on—I didn't care about anything. The only thing I never took was heroin, because I've never seen heroin. But if it was in front of me, I guarantee I would've taken it. And acid was never in front of me, so I never took acid. We'd just go to Tim's house or get blankets and pillows and all kinds of stuff and go to the beach for the night.

With all the peer pressure to stick to one group of friends and her own insecurities, Sandi basically insulated herself from everyone else except Tim.

We'd get high all the time and ditch school. But still, he became very physically abusive and verbally abusive, and one time he hit one of my friends. She wanted her jacket back that he was wearing, and he didn't want to give it back 'cause he was cold, so he smacked her in the face. He just went poof. And she just took off running. She ran that way and he ran in the house, 'cause it was in front of his house. I was standing out there, I didn't know which way to go. I couldn't get home, 'cause he had to drive me home. So I was confused on which way to go, and I took off and went to him, 'cause he was like out of control—he was in a rage, he was slamming doors, throwing furniture around. I tried to calm him down and stuff. And then my friend shined me on because she didn't think it was right that I went after my boyfriend instead of her. So I never saw her again. She was history.

My parents kept asking me why I didn't have other friends, but I shined them on. I was tired of their complaints. They complained all the time—about my grades, whatever—but I didn't do anything about them. I told them, "I am not in school for an education, I'm there for a social life." They were like, "We wish you would do better in school," you know, that kind of thing. And I would just be like, I would just sit and stare at the wall, you know. I started becoming this walking zombie.

Soon marijuana wasn't even getting me high anymore. It was like bringing me to a normal state. I was still smoking it every day, even though it didn't do anything. And I was drinking a lot—beer, California Coolers, vodka. Then speed and cocaine every once in a while. Also downs, Quaaludes. My boyfriend, Tim, gave it all to me; I didn't have to buy anything. I'm not sure how he got it. I didn't ask 'cause I didn't care.

**Reflecting her zombie-like state, Sandi's manner of dress changed dramatically.**

I would wear short leather miniskirts with zippers on the sides and black fishnets and black spike beads with studs on 'em, and red lipstick and my whole face with makeup, and fishnet shirts with black bras underneath, and that's how I would go to school. I looked like I belonged on Hollywood Boulevard or something, not in school, but that's how I dressed. See, it was like something was wrong with me and I knew something was wrong. Now, I didn't know what was wrong with me, and all I wanted to do was be happy. That's what I knew. That's the only thing I knew. I just wanted to be happy. There were times when I just felt like I wanted to die. But my biggest dream now was just to be happy. And I had no idea that drugs and happiness were incompatible.

I guess finally my parents saw something was up, maybe when they saw how I was dressing, so they asked me to go to this group thing, this therapy thing with them, and I said I wouldn't go. They went without me. And then they asked me again, and I said yes. This girl I knew, Lilith, was there with her parents. She was going through, I guess, the same sorts of things I was. So I didn't mind going. I liked it there for some reason. It was like, the kids were talking about things that were bothering them, and I still couldn't talk about what was bothering me, but it felt like I was safe. I was in a good place. Some of the times I went there I was high and some of the times I wasn't. I'd get high at school, or before, and then go, 'cause this was like seven o'clock at night.

One of the things the parents were learning at this group was to kick their kids' butts—not physically, but to be disciplined. You know, kick them out of the house if necessary, that sort of thing. But my parents couldn't do it. They tried to, but it didn't work. I mean, they wouldn't kick me out of the house. They could never see kicking their own child out of their house. And what happened was, every week at the kids' group—see, the kids and the parents would meet separately—they'd try to get you back into, like, motivation about life and goals that you want to achieve, and, like, every week my short-term goal was to go to school. And soon they saw, like, a pattern of this, and the guy who ran the place started asking, you know, "Why aren't you going to school?" And I said, "Because I'm getting high." It was like I finally didn't care. "Yeah, I'm getting high." And see, when I looked at people around me, it was like everybody's getting high, you know, this is what everybody's doing, and life is miserable and some people cope with it better. I thought everybody was miserable. I thought life was depressing; I thought life was just horrible, and I thought everybody was using as much as me, or more, so I was okay. There was no question in my mind whether I was a drug addict, because I didn't know really what a drug addict was. I couldn't have been. The only thing I knew was the bum on Skid Row. So that wasn't me. I wasn't on Skid Row, and I was not a bum. I dressed nice—at least, I thought I dressed nice; I have a nice house, and I drive a car which my parents have given me, and, you know, I'm not no bum. So I wasn't an addict.

But I really thought life sucked. Life was the pits. You know, I had a boyfriend who beat me up and I didn't understand it. I mean, one time when I was staying at his house when his parents were on vacation, I was laying outside in the pool in my bathing suit. And I came in the house and I went into his room to change my bathing suit, and he came behind me and started hitting me with a belt. I had like welts all over my back. I didn't do anything wrong. I just walked in the house to change my bathing suit. So I didn't understand what was going on, yet I was too scared to tell anybody. And I think my friends knew what was going on, 'cause he would come up to me at school when I was walking down the hall looking for someone, and he would slam me into the locker. I took this from him, but see, it also wasn't totally his fault that he was doing this because I didn't care about myself anymore. The drugs had made me not care. It was just like, "Well, if he's gonna hit me, then I must deserve it, I'm worthless, you know, and this is what's gonna happen."

I didn't care about myself, my boyfriend was hitting me, life sucked, drugs weren't getting me high anymore, and this was, like, all towards the end of the school year. I was running away from home, and I was running to him and he was gonna take care of me, yet I knew somehow he was gonna hurt me really bad. He was graduating that year, and I went to this amusement park with him and a bunch of friends for the night. This is weird, 'cause I just found this out from my mom a couple weeks ago, but that night he gave me some weed to smoke, and I was smoking it, and all of a sudden everything started flashing and ringing in my ears and I was moving in slow motion. He'd laced the weed, and I didn't know at the time that he did it. I didn't even know this till he got sober. I was going, "Tim, Tim, it's doing it again, it's doing it again." I thought my body was fucked up, and he's like, "Don't worry about it, just relax and calm down." And I was standing there in line, and everything was flashing black and white and I was like moving in slow motion, holding onto the railings; my legs felt like noodles. Two of my friends, these guys I knew, who happened to be there were like, "Are you okay?" Tim was in the bathroom and they saw me. I'm like, "Yeah, I'm okay," and in my head, my head's telling me, "If you go on that roller coaster you're gonna die." I passed out in line when he came back, and he had to carry me back to some bench or something, and, like, the rest of the evening was like a dream, it was like fog. I didn't even remember it.

What I found out a couple weeks ago was that that night he called my parents, 'cause they were always in a feud—him against them. It was like a tug of war and I was stuck in the middle—this drugged-out zombie: Who's gonna get me first? Who's gonna take control of me and who's gonna be able to have me? That night, he called my parents and he said, "Sandi's with me and you're never getting her back." Now, I didn't even know that till a couple weeks ago, so now I know for sure that he laced that weed. I think he thought that, now that I was smoking weed that was laced with PCP, I was his, 'cause he saw the way I reacted to it; I was just like nothing. And the next morning, I was like, "Did we go there? What did we do?" I didn't remember anything. I knew I'd passed out, but from that point on, the rest of the night was kinda like, "Did we really stay the whole night there, or was that a dream?" And he was like, "Yeah, we were there." And so after that, from that night on, I was staying with him for like two weeks. I wasn't at home and my parents were like worried about me. The cops were coming all the time. You know, I was underage. He was eighteen and I was seventeen and that's underage, so they could've got him for statutory. So the cops were coming to his house and they were hiding me and his parents were freaking out. And so I started staying next door with his neighbor and watching their kids; the police were getting too close and Tim was getting scared—he had warrants out for him for tickets. So he said, "You need to go home now, and in a couple weeks maybe you can come back." And I was like, "Okay." I'd been smoking his PCP pot, and I didn't even know it was laced, so I was completely gone. Whatever someone said, that's what I did.

I was just a total zombie. I was like, "Okay, I'll go home now." And so I called my parents and asked them if I can come home, and they said yeah. And I was sitting in my room in the middle of the floor, just sitting there, staring at the carpeting, and five men walked in, and these men looked familiar but I didn't know who they were. It turns out they were from that group we'd gone to that my parents were still going to. And they had come to take me to the hospital. My parents are freaking out and stuff. My mom was like, "There's something wrong with our daughter, and I'm putting her in a hospital, and you don't have to be here if you don't want to." 'Cause my dad was like, "How can I take her to a hospital when I said she can come home?" And my mom goes, "Well, you don't have to be here when we do this." And so they took me. They told me I was going for, like, drug tests, and it was so strange, because I was like, "Well, I'm gonna show them I'm not using drugs," but here I was using drugs, and they said, "If you're clean then you won't have to stay," and I was like, "Cool," and I really believed in my head I wasn't doing drugs. And we're driving and we're driving, and I'm like, "Where's the place." And it was like I was in a stunt car; the doors didn't open or anything, 'cause they thought I was gonna run, and so they got me to the hospital, and the guy who runs the group was there, and he told me to tell my parents that I understood that I was going to a hospital for tests. I had no idea what I was talking about, I was still high from the night before. So I went up to my parents, and they're like bawling, they are crying hysterically and I'm like, "It's okay, I really understand." I was like, "Don't worry, I really understand, it's okay." I had no idea what I was doing. But I think my subconscious mind might have known that I was staying. 'Cause everytime I walked down the hall with the counselor I kept turning around and walking back. I kept going and giving my parents a hug. Then I'd walk back down the hall and I'd turn around and go back.

I went into the hospital for three and a half months, but the second week I was there I left. Me and this girl AWOL'd through the air conditioner. We broke out. We pulled it out of the wall. Someone told us that the air conditioners come off. And we got out, 'cause it was just like a wall unit that pulled out of the wall and there was just the air on the outside. So we pulled the air-conditioning thing out, and we're on this ledge and we jumped off, and I fell on my hip and we're running down the street, and we're running to the freeway 'cause we're gonna run all the way home—and it was about probably twenty miles. I mean, it was, like, we were stupid, 'cause we would of got picked up. But we didn't because there was a car sitting on the freeway ramp, and there was music coming from it. And my friend Tammy goes, "Wow, let's go over to that car," and I said, "No way." I was like scared someone was gonna jump out with a knife or something, you know, and she's going, "Come on." 'Cause we had already met a whole bunch of other weirdos that kept saying they'd give us rides and wanted to give us money. And Tammy's like, "We just AWOL'd from a hospital, we don't have time, da-da-da." And I'm like, "Shut up. You don't go around telling people that." And so we saw this car, and went over to the car, and we looked inside and no one was there and the motor was on. And I was like, "Whoa, this is weird." She goes, "Get in." And I said, "I ain't drivin' if we're stealing this car." She goes, "I don't have a license." So I get in and I go to turn the key and there's no key. The car was already hotwired. So we took off, and I was like, "Cool, nrrrrr." And the whole time the car was like fucked up. The wheel was, like, wobbling. I'm like, "Tammy, we're gonna crash." You know, I'm like doing seventy-five on the freeway, and the car's going "n-n-n-n." Like we're gonna get stopped for drunk driving or something. Like I was out to prove I wasn't an addict. That's what I believed I was doing. I was still in a really bad fog, and I was like, "I'm gonna prove I'm not an addict."

When we AWOL'd, we did not get loaded. We went to Tim, of course, my boyfriend. It was just for the night, 'cause he had been in a hospital and he was started to get like, "Uh-oh, what's best for her," 'cause he knew about the hospital, and it's like once you're in the hospital and you get loaded again . . . So what happened was, the car crashed a block away from his house; the tire popped off and flew over the car, and that's what was making the car go like "r-r-r-r" all the time. It was amazing it went as far as it did. So then we got to his house and his parents were there, so we went to go find Tammy's boyfriend, but her boyfriend was put in jail for drugs. So that night we stayed at my friend Connie's house—all of us, 'cause her parents were out of town. So we stayed the night, and we didn't get high, and they brought us back to the hospital the next day. Just like that. We found out the hospital tried to call our parents, but my parents they didn't get hold of, because they weren't home. And they called the police and stuff. But they didn't know how far we—they thought we were on foot, and then they thought that my boyfriend came and picked us up, and we're like, "No, we stole this car," and they're like, "We don't believe you."

But here's another weird thing: When we were walking towards the doors and stuff, going back into the hospital, there was like a feeling, like so powerful, like it was bringing us in without us thinking. 'Cause we were still thinking, "We're gonna get out of this, and let's go dancing tonight." You know, that's what we really wanted, and we walked around the hospital two times 'cause we couldn't decide, and we were walking in silence. And it was kind of like, like a powerful feeling, like it was a magnet. I think there was a part of me that really knew this was the answer. I stayed there for three and a half months, and I fought through the whole program; I didn't want it, you know, and I didn't want to change. "I'll stop using drugs but I'm not gonna change, and I'm not gonna let go of my boyfriend." I didn't have any problem letting go of my other friends, 'cause they were letting go of me anyway. But not Tim. That was it. He just had this power over me, and I thought I really loved him. I destroyed my family. I was destroyed.

He was calling me and bringing me presents, and they wouldn't let him see me, though. He was the only visitor I couldn't have. 'Cause my parents had an idea that he was abusive to me. And I started sharing that at the hospital, you know, 'cause I had groups with girls sharing that kind of thing. I said, "Oh, well, my boyfriend does that," and they're like, "Don't you see anything wrong with that?" I'm like, "No. He loves me, you know. He wouldn't do something bad to me, you know." So my mind was really distorted by the time I got to the hospital. I mean, my thinking was just like not rational at all.

After three and a half months in the rehab hospital, Sandi was ordered placed in a halfway house in a nearby town. Most of the other girls there had also been ordered by the court to live there.

There was two houses, and I was there for a week. I was supposed to be there longer, but the first night we went to a football game and someone gave me a beer. So I drank the beer and I thought, "Cool, I'm gonna learn to control my drinking now, you know, this is how they're gonna show me." And that's what my mind was really telling me; actually, it was just playing tricks on me. So the next two days I didn't get high or loaded, and then I started going to the school that all the other girls there went to; it was a public high school, and me and this girl started going, 'cause she was new in the house too. And I don't think she really gave a shit about being sober. And we went to school and we registered for all our classes, and then we took off. This was supposed to be my senior year. And we left right after; we didn't even go to the classes. And I wanted to get high really bad, and so did this girl. So I called the hospital to talk to my counselors, and I said, "I feel like getting high, you know, da-da-da-da." They said to go back to school. I said, "I can't do that," and they said, "Well, then don't get high. But you need to go back to school." And I said, "Okay," and I hung up the phone and I didn't go back. And as we're walking down the street, this workman comes by and he asks us where we're going. We're saying, "Down the street to the liquor store," so he gave us a ride there, and he goes, "Well, you know, what do you guys want? I'll buy it for you, I don't care." And he brought us into the liquor store, and we picked out two four-packs of California Coolers each, and he was smoking weed with us in his truck. So we're sitting on the grass along the boulevard, and we're sitting down there with this dude and we have no idea who it is, and we're just drinking away and smoking weed right there, you know, and it was like no big deal, just passing these joints around and drinking. Eventually, he had to leave, 'cause his lunch break was over. So this guy's buying us booze and leaving us. So we didn't care, you know. And then this guy comes up to us and asks us, "Hey, you know, do you have any money to get some dope?" This guy looked too clean for what he was wearing; he kinda like looked like a narc. And like at first we were like, "Yeah, we have, you know." He's, "I can get you anything, anything you want. I mean, you name it, I'll get it for you, anything." And he kept saying "anything." And we're like, hmmm. So we're like, "Okay, come back here tomorrow, you know, and we'll tell you what we want. We'll meet you here at two o'clock tomorrow." We couldn't get this guy away from us. And so he goes, "Okay, okay, you promise you'll be here?" We're like, "Yeah, yeah, yeah."

The next day, for school, I didn't even bring my books. When I got out of the hospital I bought a whole new wardrobe of clothes to start like over again, clothes that weren't black. It was like a different style of dressing. But I still had a few things that were what I used to wear. And the next day, I wore black leather pants, black leather boots, a black and red leather shirt, and a black purse, and that's how I went to school. I got on the bus and I thought I was cool, you know, and this girl gets on the bus and goes, "What're you doing? Are you going to school today?" I said, "Are you crazy? I'm not going to school." She goes, "What're you doing?" I go, "I'm gonna go get high." And she said, "Oh, okay." So then she took her books and threw 'em out the bus door before it took off, threw 'em in a bush. And this other guy that was with us said, "What are you guys doing? I want to go, you know. You're not going to school, can I go with you guys?" We're like, "Yeah." So it was the three of us, and we got on the bus. We only had a bus pass for a certain bus line down there, so we ended up downtown, but we didn't have any money so we decided, well, let's try and sell my gold here. I was gonna sell all my gold jewelry to go get high. Weird, huh?

When we got off the bus, turns out we were right down there on Skid Row with the bums. As I said earlier, I did not consider myself an addict because I wasn't on Skid Row. Well, that day I was down there and I was trying to sell my gold to get money for dope. This guy starts following us around, and he was trying to sell us his dope, but we didn't have any money. He knew we were trying to go sell my jewelry, so he followed us around, and we were talking. He was introducing us to people. He brought us into some topless strip club or something and introduced us to the guys in there. I was seventeen years old. We felt really strange in there, but it was like, walking on the street, I felt like I belonged there. It was like, these were my friends, which is really sad, because we looked out of place down there—yet I felt totally comfortable. I felt like this was home. I can remember walking down the streets and not being scared of anybody, which normally you would be down there, 'cause I've been down there in my sobriety just to see where I actually was, and it was like I was only down there for the day but I remember how comfortable I was.

We couldn't hock my jewelry 'cause I didn't have my driver's license. We're sitting on the corner and we're smoking this guy's stuff. What happened was, he said, "Well, fuck it, let's smoke it anyhow." So we're all sitting there smoking it and the cops pull up. I was so gone, I didn't even hear what anyone was saying. They're all, "Throw it out, throw it out, throw it out." And I took a hit. And the cops are walking towards us, and they're asking us what we're doing here, you know, and we said, "Well, we got to school late and we were getting out early today, for a shortened day, and so we were gonna come down and go shopping, but we got off at the wrong stop."

So we're saying that, and he goes, "Well, what are your names, you know, can we see your ID?" And it was, like, me and Nikki didn't have any ID because yesterday was our first day of school and we didn't get our ID's; we were supposed to get 'em that day, but we weren't there. And the guy we were with showed 'em his ID and then they started asking us, "Where are you guys really from, da-da-da." We told 'em we were in a placement, and this one cop goes, "Is that yours over there?" He was pointing to this joint we'd thrown on the ground when we saw them. I was like, "No, no, I don't get loaded, I don't party. We're in a placement for drug and alcohol rehabilitation," and all that kind of stuff. So they said, "Come with us." So we all piled in the car and they took our purses and they emptied everything. And they didn't find drugs 'cause we didn't have any drugs, but they took us each into this little place where kids who ditched school get put, so we didn't get booked or anything. And the guy took me in his office and he sat me down and said, "If I see you down here one more time I'm throwing you in the hall." Meanwhile, they give you this like rice thing to eat and an apple for lunch, and I didn't like that; I didn't even want to try that stuff, so I'm like blinking my eyes and flirting with the officers. "Can I please have another apple?" Miss Cutesy now. They said, "Okay." And one of the guys is all, "Hmmmm," and this other cop comes up and goes, "It's okay, it's okay, I brought her in, she can have another apple." No one else got a second apple. It works with cops too.

Then the guy from the placement picked us up. We knew we were busted now. They had this big encounter-group thing and everybody was raggin' on us and screamin' at us, "How can you do this? Everybody ditches school, but you should talk about it, da-da-da-da." So that night me and this girl and this guy planned to split; we were gonna leave. But Nikki never showed up; I don't know what happened. To this day, I don't know what happened. But me and this other guy split. We were walking down the highway and it started raining, and we had like bags and stuff. There was a bridge overcrossing and we went under it to stay out of the rain. And he like passed out right away and I'm sitting there going, "Oh, my God, what am I doing here?" It's like I had a moment of clarity: "What are you doing here? Why did you go to that hospital? Why did you come here? Now you're back where you started again."

I started hitting this guy—just kind of went crazy, just hitting him. I said, "Screw this, I'm going to call somewhere." I went to the telephone and I called all the counselors from the hospital and some people that worked at the hospital. They all said to call my mom and dad. So I took a risk and I called my parents, 'cause it was like at this point I wanted to stay somewhere. They picked me up and took me home, and I was home for a week. Then I went back into the hospital, 'cause that's when I really started taking my dad's Valiums. I was there for another month, and after that I went to a women's recovery home.

At this point, I still have not let go of Tim. I didn't have any contact with him, but I did not let go of him. So when I was at this recovery home I couldn't call anyone or talk to anyone for thirty days. But the second month I could make calls and I started talking to him, and it started gettin' real appetizing to see him. It probably was like about three or four months since I'd seen him. And he's like, "Baby, I love you so much, things are gonna change, da-da-da. I'm trying to stay sober, da-da-da." Giving me this whole line of stuff. So that day, when I decided I was gonna go meet him, I was just gonna go meet him for lunch and we weren't allowed to do that; at this house, we weren't allowed to meet any of our friends for lunch or anything. But it was on the honor system and they let you out for two hours every day. You weren't allowed to go see anyone you knew; you're allowed to go shopping, go to the mall, stuff like that.

So I decided I was going out and I was gonna go see him. So I went and I met him and he took me to lunch.

This was at a place about a mile from the halfway house. He goes, "I'm not taking you back there," and I said, "You have to." He says, "No, no, I'm not going to. You're gonna stay with me now." In a way, he was kidnapping me. What happened was, we were on his motorcycle and he started heading back to the place and he keeps saying, "I'm not taking you back there. I refuse to take you back there." He gets off the freeway and turns around and starts going back towards his house—I don't know, about ten or fifteen miles. He knew someone who was out of town, I guess, that lived near him, but in the boondocks, in a real secluded house by itself, on the top of this hill. I never even knew it was there. And he took me there. And it was like that's where I was living now. Someplace I had no idea. I hated being with him, I hated being with him. Before I saw him I wanted to be with him so bad, but I'd grown so much emotionally through the program. Even though I'd gotten loaded here and there, I knew I'd learned a lot. And when I finally got to see him, it was like I didn't even want him to touch me. I didn't want to be near him or anything. So I got high. And I felt okay with him when I was high.

I was with him for about two and a half weeks. He wouldn't let me leave the house; he like locked up the house and there was no way for me to leave. He didn't have a car, all he had was his motorcycle now. There was, like, nowhere for me to go. Sometimes he would leave me there for a couple minutes and go down to the store or something, and he told me that if he found out that I was calling anybody, he was really gonna hurt me. I believed he'd do it too, 'cause he'd hurt me before. I didn't know it then, but I definitely believe now that there was something wrong with this guy.

That whole time, I made sure I was high when I was with him, because I could not stand to be around him. All I had was the clothes I was wearing, and I was too scared to call my parents and tell them what happened. I ended up getting hold of one of my ex-boyfriends from ninth grade. I looked his phone number up in the book when Tim was out; he was trying to sell like health foods door-to-door; I was too scared, too weird, too high, too fucked up to call the police or anything. You know, 'cause at the time, it didn't even seem too weird. So I called this guy and he said, "Well, tell me where you are." I say, "I don't know where I am." I didn't know what street I was on, and I didn't know where this house was. He said to go outside and look at the street sign and call him tomorrow at this same time and he'd come and get me. And at that moment Tim was walking in the door and I hung up. I never called him back.

Our room consisted of a mattress on the floor and beer boxes for end tables. And that was real different for me, because I had everything I always wanted at home. So I tried to make the room look pretty. I, like, put weeds in a cup; that was pretty to me, 'cause there was nothing else around. I remember, he used to go off on little things. I was in the room one time with the radio blaring and I was like having a good old time by myself, dancing around the room. I was like totally high, and he came running in and slammed the door and goes, "What do you think you're doing? Are you some kind of a teenager?" And my head was going, "But I'm seventeen, I don't understand what he's talking about," so it really freaked me out. I turned the radio lower. I was paranoid; every time he would go off I didn't know whether he was gonna come to me or hit me. One time, he did hit me.

**Believing that Sandi had run away from the halfway house of her own volition, her parents and the house directors did not call the police; they had given up. Sandi, meanwhile, was too afraid and confused to call the police, the house, or her parents when she had the opportunity.**

See, it was like after he took me from there and after I started getting high, I didn't care. I was living in fear of being beaten, but then it was, like, I was getting high again and it was okay. When you're addicted, once you start . . . I'll always like getting high, even though I shouldn't. I'm an addict. It was, like, I felt so bad for doing it 'cause I knew, so I kept doing more and more and more to turn off those feelings, to cover it up. So what happened was, we threw a party at the house, and Tim invited all these people, and a lot of my old friends showed up. I was like obliterated, I was so high. One of these friends in particular knew I had split from that place, or thought I had split or something. She told my mom that I was staying there, but she never came and got me because she thought I was there on my own will; she thought I wanted to be there. She thought I left the recovery house, and they were at the point where they didn't know what to do with me anymore, because I had been through the hospital twice and been to two recovery homes by now, so they were just kind of shining me.

One day I was laying there and my old friend Tammy's phone number just kind of flashed through my mind. So I called her and she says, "Well, let me talk to Tim when he gets home." I gave her the phone number to call back. And he was, like, pissed, but it was Tammy, so it was okay. And I convinced him to let me stay at her house. He said, "Are you gonna run on me, da-da-da?" I said, "No, no, no, I promise I won't." It was like, "I'll be good, don't worry, I'm not gonna run." That night she took me to one of those meetings that I'd gone to a long time before, when they put me in the hospital for the first time. And the news had already spread that I was using again. Tammy said she wasn't, but like every couple weeks she'd go and get loaded. But she took me there 'cause she saw me falling apart in front of her eyes, and all the people there knew I was gone again, so when I showed up there, they were like, "Do you want to go home? Do you want to go home?" And I said, "Yes, but they're not gonna take me this time." So they said, "Well, maybe they will if we talk to them," and I told them what happened that two weeks, and they said, "Well, we'll get you home, you'll be okay."

My parents let me home, but I had to stay in my brother's room. They locked me out of my room 'cause they thought I was just coming home to get clothes and items that I needed. Every morning I could go into my room and get something I needed to wear, and then they'd lock it up again. And every day I had to go to this rehab house, where the counselor in charge had complete control over my life; she decided who I got to see, who I could eat lunch with, all that stuff. For the first couple weeks Tim would come over to our house and start banging on the door. "Let me in, I have to see her, I have to talk to her"—totally like harassing us. He was in front of the house every time we wanted to leave. I couldn't even step on my front porch because he would be there. Meanwhile, I'm trying to stay sober now, going to this rehab place and really trying, really sticking with the program. But he made it tough, 'cause shit, it's hard enough trying to quit without some maniac harassing you all the time. They ended up getting a restraining order, but it took a long time 'cause they couldn't prove anything; there were no other witnesses or something. Even when we got the restraining order, he didn't really care, he would come over anyhow. We had to keep going down to the police, go through the lawyers, have them call his lawyer, tell them he better stop or he's going to jail, da-da-da. To this day he still harasses me. There's no proof he's doing it, yet I know that it's him. It's like, sometimes I'll come home and I'll feel like someone's staring and watching me; I'll have that feeling and I know it's true. I mean, I believe he loved me in that sick way. I believe he really loved me, but I believe he didn't know how to show me the right way to love. It's like a sickness. But I believe somewhere in his heart he loved me. And I know that somewhere in my heart I loved him. I am scared of him, though. I'm really scared of him. My parents left one weekend, and I came home and on the newspaper was written all over.

"Fuck you bitch. I know you still love me, you should be mine."

Not long after she entered the rehab program, Sandi started going out with another boy—a sober one.

This just shows how sick I was. The first couple times I went out with him I went into the counselor's office and I said, "He doesn't love me." And she said, "Why?" I said, "'Cause he doesn't hit me." And it was like from there till now I've grown so much. I got loaded once in between, and I believe I got loaded because I started dealing with all these heavy issues, with being abused and stuff, and then I left for the weekend with my friend. All that pain was just starting to come out, all the stuff I never dealt with except to get high. I just didn't even think and just got loaded. And then after that, I've been clean ever since. I get along really well, really well. I'm working in the recovery hospital right now. I'm dealing with adults right now, and I'm starting to work with adolescents in a couple of weeks.

I feel like I've been through a lot more than most kids my age. And I'm real observant now about the way people act, and I know a lot of my actions and I see them in others, so I can call them on it. Now, I don't even do half the things I used to do; I don't manipulate men the way I used to, and I talk about feelings, and I don't stuff the feelings inside, 'cause when I first got sober I started really heavily self-destructing. I used to try to hurt myself. I have a scar on my thigh from a cigarette burn I did myself. And I have marks on my arms where I just picked the skin off with my fingernails.

The drugs were gone and I knew I couldn't get high anymore, but I was hurting so bad inside. For the first month and a half when I was in the rehab, I didn't know how to talk, I didn't know how to express feelings, I didn't know how to get angry. I mean, it was like I was sad all the time. All I did was sit and stare at the wall. I showed no emotion except I looked like a totally depressed zombie. And I was in so much pain that I would just carve on myself. And that was a way of making the pain physical. It's like, while I was doing it I wouldn't even feel it. Not till afterwards. It was another way of hiding the pain—that's what I've learned. But I don't self-destruct anymore, and I'm like totally different. I don't dress anything like I used to, and I don't have that big judgment on people on their outward appearance, which I used to. It used to be, "What are you wearing, you know, and maybe I'll be your friend."

All I know is, drugs and alcohol brought me to a point of my life I thought I'd never be at. I thought I was like everybody else. I thought I was just an ordinary teenage kid. I didn't know there was something wrong, and I didn't know it was drugs and alcohol. You know, it's like if I want to feel like being a spastic and run around in circles like a twelve-year-old, that's okay. 'Cause I was never a little girl. And it's okay to be one now. And I don't care what other people are gonna think of me. If they think I'm childish, that's okay, 'cause my friends know me, and if someone wants to take the time to know me, then that's okay with me. I mean, I really feel like I skipped over my childhood. At twelve years old all I wanted to do was be a sex goddess for men. It's like, where did I play with dolls and where did I have the little girl things? I don't remember doing that, and now I wish I had done those things because I think they're what little girls need to do, just like little boys need to do their things. I think children deserve to be children. And I have no idea where I got in my head that I wanted to be a sex goddess for these guys. That's what I wanted to be, that was like my biggest dream, to be a stripper or call girl. I just thought it was glamorous and classy.